The
Science and Art
Of
Living A Longer
And
Healthier Life

By
CARL E. BARTECCHI, M.D.
and
ROBERT W. SCHRIER, M.D.

Foreword by Richard D. Lamm
Governor of Colorado (1975-1987)
Quotations sourced by
Barbara Lindley Schrier

EMIS, INC.
Medical Publishers
P.O. Box 1607, Durant, OK 74702-1607

toll free: 1-800-225-0694
e-mail: saleemis@emispub.com

ISBN: 0-929240-80-4

Publisher's Note
The ideas, procedures, and suggestions contained in this book are not intended as a substitute for consulting with your physician.

Printed in the United States of America

Foreword

Proust once observed that "the real voyage of discovery is not in seeking new lands but seeing with new eyes." Carl Bartecchi and Robert Schrier direct us to look at health with new eyes. Health, they suggest, is both an art and a science; and it takes an understanding of both to live a longer and healthier life. This is important to both individuals and public policy.

A nation's health has more to do with its lifestyle and habits than the quality of its health care system. Without casting aspersions on the brilliance of U.S. medicine (which has saved one desperately important to me), we know clearly that your best doctor is yourself. We can avoid many more diseases than we can cure. Our habits are more important than our hospitals. The authors know the most valuable thing they can do for the public is to educate people on what they can do for themselves. They recognize that "medicine" and "health" are related but are not Siamese twins.

National polls confirm that "health" is one of the American public's most important priorities. But how does one achieve a long and healthy life? The authors inform us of a wide variety of simple things we can do for ourselves. These are obvious but still too often overlooked.

Victor Fuchs has written:

The greatest current potential for improving the health of the American people is to be found in what they do and don't do to and for themselves. Individual decisions about diet, exercise, and smoking are of critical importance; and collective decisions affecting pollution and other aspects of the environment are also relevant.

As a public policy maker, I feel that my patient is society. It is important to distinguish between a doctor's role and a public policymaker's. Public policy must, by definition, ask macro questions, such as "How do we keep a society healthy?" and "How do we invest limited funds to buy the most health?"

I started asking these questions when I was in the Colorado legislature. I could not understand why there was (and is) an inverse correlation in the developed world between health spending and health.

The U.S., Canada, and Germany spend the most on health care; yet they have (generally) the worst health statistics. Japan spends the least and has the best. I was told that the Japanese recognized that getting people jobs and increasing living standards will buy far more health for a country than having a health care system.

The U.S. Department of Health and Human Services estimates that, of the 30 years that have been added to human life expectancy this century, only five of those years are due to clinical medicine. We all must learn better what we can do for ourselves. With all their medical training, the authors still remind us that our health depends more on ourselves than on them.

Medicine is a profession, but health policy is a public policy choice. Our government pays more than 40 percent of health care costs. Health care costs are bankrupting more and more businesses and are dampening needed wage increases. Medicare is fast heading toward bankruptcy. Our aging bodies can thus bankrupt our children. Inquiring minds increasingly ask "How do we keep a society healthy?"

This argument is timeless. The ancient Greeks had two theories concerning health: one symbolized by the goddess Hygeia and the other by the god Aesculapius. Hygeia was the guardian of health, but her role was to symbolize the belief that people would stay in good health if they lived according to reason. She represented moderation in lifestyles, not treatment of the sick. Aesculapius, in contrast, was concerned with identifying the cause of disease and the treatment of the sick.

These divergent views of health have never been resolved and remain a key issue today, one that will grow during the next 10 years. Dr. Bartecchi and Dr. Schrier brilliantly bridge these two aspects of health. Both are scholars in allopathic medicine; yet both recognize that we currently do not inform the public enough on how people can take care of their own health. Their book is filled with useful and practical suggestions on how individuals, families, and societies can best maintain health.

The authors, thus, have risen above the excellence of their own specialties and have looked at the big picture. They are concerned with both medicine and health and have given us a practical guide to use in our daily lives.

Richard Lamm,
Governor of Colorado
1975-1987

Dedication

To our wives, Kay and Barbara, who continue to help us live longer, healthier, and happier lives.

Acknowledgements

The authors wish to recognize Shirley Artese and Kay Bartecchi for expert technical assistance. We appreciate the insightful and thought-provoking quotations provided by Barbara Lindley Schrier.

About The Authors

Carl Bartecchi and Robert Schrier are a unique physician team that has worked together for more than a decade in several health care and educational areas. Dr. Bartecchi, a pre-eminent practitioner of internal medicine for more than 30 years, has been recognized nationally, having received both the prestigious American College of Physicians' Ralph O. Claypoole Memorial Award and Colorado's Distinguished Internist Award of the American College of Physicians. Bartecchi is also Clinical Professor of Medicine at the University of Colorado School of Medicine.

Dr. Schrier has been Professor and Chairman of the Department of Medicine at the University of Colorado for 20 years. His department's training program ranks among the best in the country. In 1996 Schrier received the Robert H. Williams Award from the Association of Professors of Medicine as the outstanding Chairman of Medicine in the country.

Although educating physicians and patients has been the continual focus of Bartecchi and Schrier, this text, *The Science and Art of Living a Longer and Healthier Life*, is written for the lay public in response to patients' requests and the need for medically sound and substantiated data. The text includes the best scientific and practical information available for individuals who desire to make reasonable efforts to extend the quality and length of their lives.

The Science and Art of Living a Longer and Healthier Life

Expert Reviewers

Richard Bakemeier, M.D., Professor of Medicine, Division of Medical Oncology, UCHSC

Robert Ballard, M.D., Associate Professor of Medicine, Division of Pulmonary Science and Critical Care Medicine, UCHSC

Blair Carlson, M.D., Clinical Professor, Department of Medicine, UCHSC

Steven Dubovsky, M.D., Professor of Medicine and Psychiatry, UCHSC

Robert Eckel, M.D., Professor of Medicine, Division of Endocrinology, UCHSC, President, North American Society for the Study of Obesity

William Hiatt, M.D., Professor of Medicine, Chief, Section of Vascular Medicine, UCHSC

Fred Hofeldt, M.D., Professor of Medicine, Chief of Endocrinology, Denver Health Medical Center

Steve Johnson, M.D., Assistant Professor of Medicine, Division of Infectious Diseases, UCHSC

Stuart Linas, M.D., Professor of Medicine, Division of Nephrology, Chief of Nephrology, Denver Health Medical Center

Steven Mostow, M.D., Professor of Medicine, Chief of Medicine, UCHSC, Columbia Rose Medical Center

Allan Prochazka, M.D., Associate Professor of Medicine and Preventive Medicine, UCHSC

Stuart Schneck, M.D., Professor of Neurology, UCHSC

Phil Wolf, M.D., Professor of Medicine, Clinical Director, Division of Cardiology, UCHSC

Table of Contents

RISK FACTORS

DISEASE PREVENTION/HEALTH AIDS

GENERAL INFORMATION

CONCLUSION

FIGURES

Introduction

Since the turn of the century, life expectancy of Americans has increased by about 30 years, from 45 to 75 years old. This significant gain can be attributed to various reasons, including health care, better nutrition, sanitation, occupational safety and housing. Unfortunately, however, large numbers of our population will not come anywhere close to the 75th year. Some individuals otherwise capable of quality years well beyond age 75 will not be able to achieve that potential.

Certainly accidents, wars, natural disasters, or the unfortunate acquisition of certain diseases can abruptly terminate life, but it has been estimated that 50 percent of premature deaths are associated with choices people make, including the abuse of tobacco, alcohol, and other toxic substances; unhealthy diets; and sedentary lifestyles. Further significant reductions in premature deaths can be accomplished by reducing environmental risks and improving access to medical treatment.

Today more than ever, scientific studies and observations indicate that almost anyone's lifespan, from almost any age as a starting point, can be extended by incorporating certain reasonable, rational, and inexpensive actions or strategies into the lifestyle. Unfortunately, there is no guarantee regarding quality of the extended period of life, but it appears that these same principles often also contribute to improved quality of extended life. Accomplishing life extension requires positive actions and definite commitments by those interested in such a long-term goal.

This discussion is directed to individuals in their mid-20s and beyond. Younger individuals tend to be preoccupied by other more pressing concerns as well as being protected by a certain feeling of immortality. Though without proof, the authors' personal feelings are that the 40th birthday appears to trigger early thoughts of "just how long the ol' bod can make it" for most people.

We all arrive in this world with a genetic makeup that has an important influence on the quality and length of our lives. In the future, genetic engineering can be expected to help improve chances for a better and a longer life; but for now, the tried and tested actions and principles that are supported by studies in the medical literature and reinforced by successful trials of large numbers of individuals are the standards to be used. The authors have taken care to avoid unreasonable or overly expensive recommendations that would not be available to the general public or that would serve to advertise or endorse products touted as capable of extending life.

The subjects of the following chapters are associated with principles or actions that have the potential to prolong life. First, however, is a look at the causes of death from two different viewpoints, those of the American Heart Association and the National Center for Health Statistics. Each lists estimated figures for the leading causes of deaths in males and females in the United States (1989).

From the 1993 Heart and Stroke Facts Statistics, Dallas, Texas, American Heart Association, 1992:

	MALES	FEMALES
1. Cardiovascular disease	456,000	486,000
2. Cancer	263,000	233,000
3. Accidents	70,000	31,000
4. Chronic obstructive pulmonary disease	48,000	36,000
5. Pneumonia/influenza	36,000	41,000
6. Suicide	24,000	6,000
7. AIDS	20,000	2,000

From McGinnis and Foege, who point out that, of the approximately 2.14 million U.S residents who died in 1990, approximately half died of particular preventable causes:

	NUMBER OF DEATHS	PERCENTAGE OF TOTAL DEATHS
1. Tobacco	400,000	19
2. Dietary factors and activity patterns	300,000	14
3. Alcohol	100,000	5
4. Microbial agents	90,000	4
5. Toxic agents	60,000	3
6. Firearms	35,000	2
7. High risk sexual behavior	30,000	1
8. Motor vehicle injuries	25,000	1
9. Illicit use of drugs	20,000	<1
Total	**1,060,000**	**49**

Further Reading

McGinnis JM, Foege WH: Actual causes of death in the United States. JAMA 1993;270.

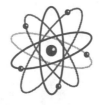

Coronary Artery Disease: The Major Cause of Death in the U.S.

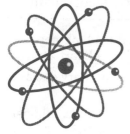

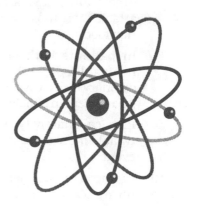

Avoid fried foods, which angry up the blood. If your stomach disputes you, lie down and pacify it with cool thoughts. Keep the juices flowing by jangling around gently as you move. Go very light on the vices, such as carrying on in society. The social ramble ain't restful. Don't look back. Something might be gaining on you.

-Satchel Paige

Facts

1. Coronary artery disease accounts for more than one-half of cardiovascular deaths and about one-third of all deaths in the U.S.

2. Heart attack is the single largest killer of American males and females.

3. This year as many as 1,500,000 Americans will have a new or recurrent heart attack and about one-third of them will die.

4. Twenty-seven percent of men and 44 percent of women die within one year of having a heart attack.

5. Persons known to be at high risk for coronary disease die 10 to 15 years earlier if they smoke.

6. It is estimated that passive smoking causes almost 40,000 heart disease deaths yearly in the U.S.

7. Men who consume a high fiber diet (especially fiber from grains) have a significantly lower risk of heart attack than those whose diet is poor in such fiber-rich foods.

8. In patients with so-called adult onset (Type II, noninsulin-dependent) diabetes mellitus, death from coronary disease is increased 200 percent in males and 400 percent in females.

9. Physical inactivity is associated with at least a twofold increase in risk for coronary artery disease events.

10. Estrogen replacement therapy in women results in up to a 50-percent reduction in the risk of developing coronary disease.

Coronary artery disease is the leading cause of death for both men and women, accounting for almost 500,000 deaths in the U.S. each year. Since 1970, however, the death rate for coronary artery disease has declined almost 50 percent due to factors relating to treatment of major risk factors.

Atherosclerosis results in blockages or hardening of coronary arteries with formation of plaque. The resultant obstruction of blood flow through the arteries causes heart attacks, heart rhythm disturbances, heart failure, and/or the numerous complications known to be associated with heart attacks. In recent years, it has become apparent that there are cardiovascular risk factors that predispose individuals to developing atherosclerosis and its subsequent complications and, thus, increase these individuals' risks of coronary artery disease. Though it is possible for people to have heart attacks and die despite having no risk factors, it is more compatible that individuals with greater numbers of risk factors and especially those with recognized problematic risk factors have the greatest danger of developing coronary disease.

Risk factors can be viewed in several ways. Some cannot be changed; these include:
- Age
- Sex
- Race
- Heredity

Others lend themselves to change and have different degrees of importance, the most important being:

- Hypertension
- Cigarette smoking
- High cholesterol levels
- Diabetes mellitus
- Enlarged heart
- Cocaine use

Actions that effectively modify these risk factors include:
- Dietary control
- Use of medications
- Quitting smoking
- Exercise
- Diabetes control
- Avoiding cocaine use

Other important modifiable risk factors include:
- Obesity
- Menopause
- Sedentary lifestyle
- Excessive alcohol consumption
- Oral contraceptive use
- Stress
- Setting at the time of a first heart attack, e.g.:
  - An individual living alone
  - A recent spousal loss or separation
  - Evidence of lack of social support

Corrective actions can effectively modify these risk factors. Protective actions include:
- The addition of estrogen
- Increased exercise
- Moderate alcohol consumption
- Enhanced HDL (good) cholesterol

Commonly seen combinations of the most important risk factors (e.g., hypertension plus cigarette smoking plus high cholesterol) can be particularly lethal. However, correcting modifiable risk factors can prevent much morbidity and mortality. The earlier that persons with modifiable risk factors are aware of and change these risk factors the greater the chance of avoiding their otherwise lethal consequences. Modifying major risk factors, such as smoking, high blood pressure, and high cholesterol levels, definitely reduces the risk of heart attack and its resulting complications. Risk factor modification, especially for patients with known coronary artery disease, improves survival rates.

Other interesting but often complex risk factors exist but are not included in this discussion other than to recognize them. These include elevated levels of fibrinogen, triglycerides, and lipoprotein (a). Elevated homocysteine levels, related to either hereditary factors or common vitamin deficiencies, can be associated with increased risk of coronary artery disease.

Recommendations
1. Assess, with the help of a physician, your cardiovascular risk factor status and re-evaluate it regularly.
2. If you smoke, STOP.
3. Eat a heart-healthy diet, specifically a diet with less fat, less meat, and more fiber-rich foods, such as fresh fruits and vegetables. Eat at least five portions of fruits and vegetables daily.

4. Maintain normal blood pressure.
5. Exercise regularly.
6. If you are overweight, reduce and aim for desirable weight.
7. Use alcohol only in moderation.
8. Postmenopausal women can benefit from estrogen replacement unless contraindications exist.
9. Never use cocaine. Even the first use of this drug can be lethal or lead to permanent cardiac damage.
10. If you are a male age 50 or older and have multiple cardiovascular risk factors, aspirin, at 75 to 325 mg, may be of value unless contraindications exist. Contraindications include poorly controlled hypertension, ulcers, and bleeding problems.
11. If you are an adult diabetic, weight loss may actually "cure" your diabetes or at least allow for better blood sugar control. A five-percent weight loss maintained over two years has been shown to prevent adult diabetes in high-risk, middle-aged individuals.

Further Reading

Twenty-seventh Bethesda Conference. Matching the Intensity of Risk Factor Management with the Hazard for Coronary Disease Events. J Am Col Cardiol, April 1996.

Heart and Stroke Facts: 1996 Statistical Supplement. American Heart Association.

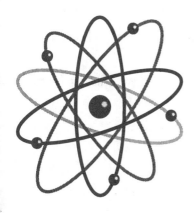

High Blood Pressure: The Silent Killer

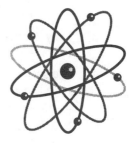

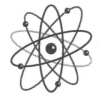

To be 70 years young is sometimes far more cheerful and hopeful than to be 40 years old.

-Oliver Wendell Holmes

Facts

1. For patients ages 60 or older, treatment of high blood pressure can reduce mortality from all causes by 12 percent, from stroke by 36 percent, and from coronary artery disease by 25 percent.

2. Studies suggest that reducing diastolic blood pressure by five to six points in all hypertensives may lower the incidence of coronary artery disease by 14 percent and strokes by 42 percent.

3. Only 24 percent of hypertensive individuals are thought to have their blood pressure under control.

4. Statistics show that only 65 percent of individuals with blood pressure at or above 140/90 mm Hg were informed of their elevated blood pressures.

5. Numerous factors can distort blood pressure readings, including location (doctor's office), instrument error, blood pressure cuff size, recent exertion, and observer error (hearing problem).

6. Many prescribed medications can cause high blood pressure.

7. In 1993 high blood pressure killed 37,520 Americans and contributed to the deaths of thousands more.

Hypertension is a common, important, and very controllable cause of stroke, heart failure, and coronary artery disease, especially in the elderly. Hypertension accelerates hardening of the arteries and is thus one of the leading risk factors for heart attack and stroke. Large numbers of people die from the heart attacks, strokes, and kidney failure caused by hypertension.

Hypertension, termed the "silent killer", is usually a symptomless disease, often discovered during routine health evaluations or screenings. Studies have shown that more than 30 percent of patients are unaware of their disease. Of those who are aware, only about one-half are under treatment; and of these, only about one-quarter are well-controlled.

It is now recognized that, as blood pressure rises from 110/80 mm Hg, the risk of cardiovascular disease increases. Repeated blood pressures at or above 140/90 fall in the hypertension range. Previously, the diastolic pressure (lower number) was considered the more important; but more recently it has been recognized that the systolic pressure, which reflects blood pressure in the arteries when the heart contracts, is more important for estimating risks of stroke and heart attack. Often systolic hypertension only is found in elderly patients.

Controlling hypertension may not require the use of medications. Lifestyle modifications can be effective to some degree in all patients; such modifications include:

- Weight reduction
- Moderate alcohol intake
- Regular physical activity
- Reduced sodium (salt) intake
- Smoking cessation

Recently, a diet low in fat and high in fruits, vegetables, low-fat dairy products, and whole grains was found to lower blood pressure effectively. Blood pressure not controlled by these measures must be treated with drugs that have proven effectiveness, especially in the elderly. In this population, drug therapy has reduced strokes by one-third and heart attacks by one-fourth. Deaths have been reduced by at least 10 percent for drug-treated patients.

Patients with hypertension must work closely with their physicians for the best results. They should have home blood pressure monitors to keep track of their own progress. Advantages of home blood pressure measurements are many, including:

- Blood pressures taken on physician/office monitors tend to be higher than those taken on home monitors
- Medications added for control of blood pressure can be monitored more closely
- Concerns about symptoms related to blood pressure highs and lows can be resolved quickly
- Stresses, activities, and/or other illnesses that affect blood pressure can be detected quickly and adjustments in therapy employed rapidly

Patients should inform their physicians about other medications they are taking that are known to elevate blood pressure. These include:

- Female hormones
- Certain arthritis medications
- Cold remedies

- Appetite suppressants
- Cocaine
- Certain antidepressant medications
- Anabolic steroids (used for muscle building)

Advantages of treating hypertension can be seen within a few years of initiating therapy and can occur even if blood pressures are not lowered to the most desirable range.

Drugs used to treat hypertension can have major and at times life-threatening complications, especially in the elderly in whom age-related changes affect the way drugs are used, altered, or eliminated from their bodies. Patients must discuss with their physicians any significant changes they detect after starting, changing, or modifying medication programs.

Recommendations

1. Even if blood pressure measurements are normal, you should have your blood pressure checked at least every two years.

2. Work closely with your physician to achieve good blood pressure control.

3. Be able to take your own blood pressure.

4. Understand your blood pressure medications. Ask your physician or pharmacist for written information about each drug. Patient-oriented information about drugs can be obtained easily.

5. NEVER stop taking blood pressure medications on your own. Stopping certain medications can result in especially severe blood pressure elevations with major complications (stroke, heart failure, or heart attack). A common cause of poor blood pressure control is patients not taking their medications because of side effects or costs of medications.

6. Avoid nondrug or natural treatments that, though often unproven, commonly are recommended for treating hypertension. These therapies, which include biofeedback, yoga, meditation, acupuncture, hypnosis, and certain fad diets, are not of the same proven effectiveness as other standard therapies and, thus, are of questionable value for effective, long-term blood pressure control.

7. The most important non-medication treatments for hypertension are smoking cessation, weight loss, salt restriction, and exercise. Among these, smoking cessation is the most important; cardiovascular complications are increased several-fold in hypertensive patients who smoke. Weight loss of as little as five to 10 percent may control blood pressure with fewer and/or lower doses of antihypertensive medications. Approximately 20 percent of hypertension patients increase their blood pressure when ingesting large amounts of salt (i.e., french fries, chips, etc.). Thus, moderate salt restriction, such as by avoiding canned goods and salty foods and by not salting foods, may help blood pressure control. This is especially true of African-Americans, the elderly, and diabetics. While exercise does not appear to decrease blood pressure as much as weight loss, it does lower the increased cardiovascular risk that is common in the hypertensive patient.

8. As high blood pressure and high cholesterol are additive with respect to cardiovascular complications, high cholesterol must be treated more aggressively in hypertensive patients than normotensive patients.

Further Reading

Fact Sheet on Heart Attack, Stroke, and Risk Factors: 1996 Cardiovascular Statistics. American Heart Association.

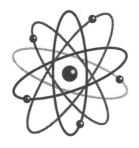

Stroke:
How to Prevent the Third Most Common Cause of Death in the U.S.

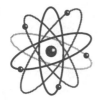

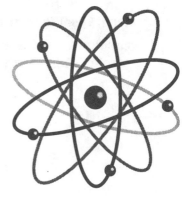

Do what you can with what you have, where you are.
                                    -Theodore Roosevelt

Facts

1. Stroke is the third leading cause of death after heart disease and cancer in the U.S.

2. Each year about 550,000 Americans suffer new or recurrent strokes.

3. The incidence of stroke more than doubles each decade after age 55.

4. High blood pressure is a major contributing factor in up to 70 percent of strokes.

5. Patients who survive an initial stroke have a recurrence rate of up to 18 percent during the following year. About 31 percent of stroke victims die within a year.

6. Stroke is the leading cause of serious long-term disability in the U.S.

7. Smokers have significantly greater risks for stroke than non-smokers.

Stroke is the third leading cause of death and the leading cause of serious disability in the U.S. Each year, half a million people, about 12 of every 10,000 Americans, suffer strokes, and about 150,000 people die from them. The risk of having a stroke increases with age, the risk being highest after age 55. The risk is higher in men until the mid-50s, when it begins to equal that of women. The risk of having a stroke also increases with family history (i.e., a close relative who has had a stroke, heart attack, or transient ischemic attack [TIA], see below).

New therapies to reduce the severity of stroke are under study but must be administered within three hours of onset of a stroke. Unfortunately, there is little in the way of effective treatment for them, but strokes can be prevented by identifying and treating people at high risk before the problem develops and by controlling risk factors. Controllable risk factors for stroke include:

- High blood pressure - Hypertension (systolic pressure greater than 140 and diastolic pressure greater than 90) may be the cause of 40 percent of strokes. Improved treatment of high blood pressure over the past 25 years has been credited with the major reduction in stroke mortality during that period

- Cigarette smoking - Smokers are 50 percent more likely to have strokes than nonsmokers; cigarette smoking predisposes to stroke by a variety of defined mechanisms. Those who quit smoking have about the same risk of stroke as nonsmokers

- Diabetes - It is estimated that diabetes can double the risk of stroke. The mechanism for this is not completely clear, though good control of diabetes and its complications should be helpful in reducing stroke risk

- Heart disease - Heart rhythm disturbances, such as atrial fibrillation, heart failure, having had a heart attack, or having had heart valve disease or valve replacement, can increase the likelihood of having a stroke. Atrial fibrillation, a common cause of irregular heart rhythm in the elderly, can increase the risk of stroke to as high as seven percent each year. Medications, including blood thinners, and surgery can significantly reduce the risk of stroke in these patients

- Vascular disease - Significant blockage of the carotid artery in the neck (greater than 70 percent narrowing) occurs in about five percent of the elderly. Even if without symptoms, the risk of stroke in these patients is three to four percent each year. This disorder can be managed by medications with or without surgery. However, depending on associated factors, as many as five percent of patients who elect surgery may have a stroke or die from the procedure itself. The physician will listen to the area over the carotid artery in the neck with a stethoscope to find evidence of blockage in the carotid artery. If found, further testing will determine the degree of blockage

- Transient ischemic attacks (TIAs) - The risk of stroke is increased in those who have had a TIA, which are reported in up to 20 percent of people who subsequently have a stroke. Aspirin and other medications have been shown to reduce the risk of stroke in patients with this condition, which is evidenced by a fleeting or transient episode of:

- Unilateral weakness
- Numbness
- Distortion of speech
- Loss of vision
- Unsteadiness
- Double vision

- Alcohol - Moderate alcohol intake (not more than two drinks daily) may be associated with a protective effect against stroke; however, heavy alcohol intake, especially in men and in those with hypertension, has been associated with an increased risk

Though many believe that type A behavior, depression, hopelessness, anxiety, psychological stress, and highly emotional life events could be risk factors for stroke, data do not confirm this.

There is some suggestion that unrecognized or "silent" strokes occur in the elderly and are manifest only by a significant decline in intellectual ability. Older individuals appear to be at greater risk of developing the more commonly recognized stroke picture.

Besides medications and surgical treatment, other approaches to avoiding stroke are recommended. These methods act by preventing or limiting further vascular lesions, controlling blood pressure, or providing nutrients or antioxidants that may prove helpful. This approach involves the maintenance of a low-cholesterol, low-fat diet with plenty of fruits, vegetables, and grains at a calorie level sufficient to maintain healthy weight. Also valuable is a daily exercise program and the avoidance of salt if patients have a tendency to high blood pressure.

Recommendations

1. Do not smoke.

2. Know your blood pressure and check it often as you age.

3. Eat at least five servings of fruits and vegetables daily.

4. Be able to recognize warning signs of TIAs.

5. Notify your physician if your heart beats irregularly.

6. Exercise daily and aim for an ideal weight.

Further Reading

Heart and Stroke Facts: 1996 Statistical Supplement. American Heart Association.

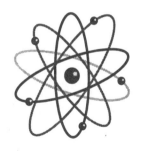

Cancer on the Rise: How to Screen for Early Detection and Treatment

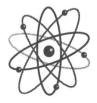

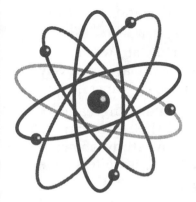

That which does not kill me makes me stronger.

-Nietzsche

Facts

1. Thirty percent of all cancers are caused by tobacco.

2. Smoking and diet may cause up to two-thirds of U.S. cancer deaths.

3. Diet, particularly high-fat and low-fiber, is a significant factor in cancer deaths in the U.S.

4. Individuals who are 40 percent over ideal weight have as high as a 55-percent greater risk of dying from cancer than those of normal weight.

5. Lung cancer is the leading cause of cancer-related deaths in both males and females in the U.S.

6. Man-made chemicals, artificial sweeteners, pesticides, and food additives are relatively insignificant or minor causes of cancer.

7. About 60 percent of human lung cancers contain mutations in the P53 tumor suppressor gene. A recent study shows a direct link between a defined cigarette smoke carcinogen (benzo [a] pyrene) and human cancer mutations.

Cancer is the leading cause of morbidity and mortality in the U.S.; and if current trends continue, it will soon become the leading cause of death. Presently more than 500,000 Americans die from cancer each year.

One-third of all Americans will eventually contract cancer. An increase in the number of cases of cancer has been recognized, but some of this is related to our population growth.

The significant growth in the number of older adults is another important factor. It has been estimated that more than 60 percent of all cancers occur after age 60 and 36 percent after age 70.

Cancer, of course, is not a single disease. There are many different forms of cancer, each with its own pattern of progression and potential for early detection, treatment, and prognosis. A relatively small number of cancers make up the majority of cancer cases:

MALES	FEMALES
Lung	Lung
Colorectal	Breast
Prostate	Colorectal
Bladder	Ovarian
Lymphoma	Uterine

Of these cancers, lung, breast, prostate, and colorectal account for more than 50 percent of all cancer deaths. Some tumors are more prevalent than might be suspected. Studies of the prostate gland during autopsy, for example, indicate that unsuspected tumors occur in 30 percent of males at age 50 and as many as 100 percent of males by age 90.

Cancers can develop from any combination of genetic, chemical, physical, or biologic insults to a body part's cells. Involved is usually a complex interplay of diet, lifestyle, and environmental factors.

Because effective treatments for many cancers are not always available, the best method appears to be prevention and/or early detection. The National Cancer Institute has estimated that early detection practices could reduce U.S. cancer mortality rates by 25 percent. Early detection is useful for cancers of the:

- Breast
- Uterine cervix
- Skin
- Mouth
- Thyroid
- Colon
- Endometrium
- Prostate
- Testicle
- Urinary bladder

Efforts to prevent cancers are useful for cancers of the:

- Lung
- Head and neck
- Skin
- Breast
- Colon
- Cervix

The opportunity to prevent cancers becomes apparent after considering that:

- About 90 percent of lung cancers among men and 79 percent among women (87 percent overall) are due to cigarette smoking

- Ninety percent of skin cancers could be prevented by protection from the sun's rays

- Seventeen thousand cancer deaths each year are related to excessive alcohol use. These are primarily cancers of the mouth and upper gastrointestinal tract and are more likely to occur in persons who both smoke and have excessive alcohol intake

- Eating a healthful diet may prevent as many as one-third of all cancer deaths. The National Cancer Institute estimates that 30,000 lives in the U.S. could be saved in the year 2000 if Americans modify their dietary habits, particularly by eating high-fiber, low-fat diets as found with increased fresh fruit and vegetable intake

- Individuals 40 percent or more overweight increase their risks of cancers of the:
  - Colon
  - Breast
  - Prostate
  - Gallbladder
  - Ovary
  - Uterus

- Epidemiological studies have shown that daily consumption of fresh fruits and vegetables is associated with decreased risks of cancers of the:
  - Lung
  - Prostate
  - Bladder
  - Esophagus
  - Colon/Rectum
  - Stomach

- High-fiber diets appear to reduce the risk of colon cancer

- High-fat diets may be a factor in the development of cancers of the:
  - Breast
  - Colon
  - Prostate

- People consuming diets high in salt-cured and smoked foods have a higher incidence of cancers of the:
  - Esophagus
  - Stomach

- Estrogen therapy in some women can increase the risk of endometrial cancer and possibly breast cancer; however, the benefits in preventing osteoporosis and heart disease are considered to outweigh the small increased risk of cancer

- Increased risks of cancers can occur from exposure to:
  - Certain tumor-killing drugs
  - Industrial agents (asbestos) and pollutants
  - Radiation
  - Gasses (radon)

Although it is known that diets rich in fruits and vegetables lower risks of developing many types of cancer, the exact agent in these foods that lowers cancer risks is not known. Numerous studies have shown that foods high in vitamins C and E, beta carotene, and other antioxidants are associated with lower risks for virtually all cancers; but specific vitamin supplements themselves have not proven effective and may potentially prove harmful. It appears that it is the actual, natural food product itself and not the antioxidant supplement that provides the protective benefit. Plant foods are loaded with bioactive substances in various mixtures and in combinations with minerals, little-studied chemicals, and numerous unknown contributors that, in some ill-defined way, protect us from many cancers. What we need to do for beneficial effects is eat a minimum of five servings of a variety of fruits and vegetables each day.

The American Cancer Society has suggested guidelines for early detection of cancer in people without symptoms. It recommends cancer-related checkups by physicians every three years for persons ages 20 to 39 and annually for those ages 40 and older. Individuals at particular risk for certain cancers or with strong family histories, however, should be evaluated more frequently. The American Cancer Society recommends that checkups include:

- Health counseling (e.g., how to quit smoking)
- Exams for cancers of the:
  - Breast
  - Uterus
  - Cervix
  - Colon
  - Rectum
  - Prostate
  - Mouth
  - Skin
  - Testes
  - Thyroid
  - Lymph nodes

That such screening is valuable is apparent, especially in the case of breast cancer. Studies suggest that, if all women ages 50 to 69 had appropriate examinations along with mammography annually, their mortality rate would decline 30 to 40 percent.

To maintain the proper perspective, it is re-emphasized that smoking and diet are the causes of about two-thirds of U.S. cancer deaths, about 25 to 40 percent and 30 percent, respectively.

Recommendations (Modified from the American Cancer Society)

FOR CANCER PREVENTION

1. Stop smoking; do not use smokeless tobacco; and avoid second-hand smoke.

2. Maintain a desirable weight.

3. Eat a varied diet with lots of high-fiber foods, such as whole grain cereal, breads, and pastas.

4. Eat fruits and vegetables, at least five servings daily.

5. Cut down on total fat intake (less than 30 percent of total caloric intake).

6. Limit alcohol consumption to no more than two drinks daily.

7. Limit consumption of salt-cured, smoked, and nitrate-cured foods.

8. Keep sun exposure to a minimum; use appropriate sunscreens.

9. Discuss needs versus risks of estrogen and progesterone replacement with your doctor.

10. Recognize and avoid occupational cancer hazards and potential radiation problems.

11. Daily aspirin appears to have preventive effects against the development of colorectal cancer. Check with your physician about the latest studies.

12. Avoid all unproven herbal supplements for prevention or treatment of cancers.

FOR BREAST CANCER SCREENING

Women ages 20 and older should do monthly breast self-examinations.

Women ages 40 to 49 should have mammograms every one to two years, at the physician's discretion, and clinical breast examinations every year. The American Cancer Society, however, recently recommended once yearly mammograms for all women in their 40s.

Women ages 50 to 69 should have annual clinical breast examinations and mammograms.

For women ages 70 and older, evidence of benefit is limited and conflicting. Physicians' recommendations should be heeded.

FOR CERVICAL CANCER SCREENING

Women ages 18 and older and those who were sexually active at younger ages should have Pap tests and pelvic examinations at least every three years and possibly yearly according to some recommendations. Regular testing can probably terminate at age 65 for women who have had regular previous screening with normal Pap smears.

FOR COLORECTAL CANCER SCREENING

Screening for colorectal cancer is recommended for all persons ages 50 and older. Annual fecal occult blood tests and sigmoidoscopy screening every three to five years currently appears reasonable, though these recommendations have changed in recent years. Earlier screening should be done for those with family histories or prior diagnoses of familial polyposis or ulcerative colitis.

FOR PROSTATE CANCER SCREENING

There is not much evidence that early detection and treatment of prostate cancer improves survival to any great extent. Large studies are presently underway to help assess the value of this. Personal physicians, possibly with help of prostate cancer specialists, can explain screening and therapeutic options available as well as the risks of evaluations and various treatments.

FOR OTHER CANCER SCREENINGS

As part of the periodic examination, physicians should examine for cancers of the:

- Skin
- Mouth
- Testes

It is helpful for patients to point out to their physicians new, suspicious, or changing lesions on any parts of their bodies.

Further Reading

Cancer Facts and Figures: 1995. American Cancer Society.

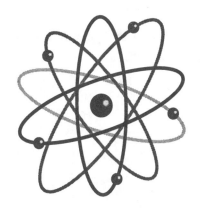

Diabetes in the Young and Old: How to Prevent Complications

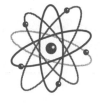

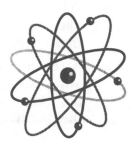

If I'd known I was going to live this long, I'd have taken better care of myself.

-Jimmy Durante

Facts

1. Diabetes is the sixth leading cause of death in the U.S. among persons ages 75 and older.

2. Estimates suggest that about 20 percent of the people ages 65 to 74 in the U.S. have diabetes.

3. It is believed that about one-half of all people with diabetes are unaware of their diagnoses.

4. People with diabetes are two to four times more likely to die from cardiovascular disease than those without diabetes.

5. A recent Harvard School of Public Health study suggests that men who smoke 25 or more cigarettes each day have roughly double the risk of developing diabetes as nonsmokers.

Diabetes is a leading cause of death and disability among Americans. About seven million people have been diagnosed with diabetes, and an equal number unknowingly have the disease. About 50,000 deaths are attributed to diabetes each year, and the disease contributes to an additional 100,000 deaths each year.

Included in the realm of diabetes mellitus and its complications are:

- High levels of sugar in the blood
- Relative or complete insufficiency of insulin, a hormone secreted by the pancreas
- Lack of response or even resistance of certain tissues to the action of insulin
- Premature development of degenerative changes in various tissues and organs
- Complications that lead to various disabling conditions and a shortened life

Patients with Type I diabetes mellitus (nine percent) have a pancreas with little or no capability of manufacturing insulin. This form of diabetes can occur at any age but most commonly is seen in young children and adolescents.

Patients with Type II diabetes mellitus (91 percent) retain some capability of producing insulin but show marked resistance or insensitivity to its action. Type II patients are often ages 40 or older and usually overweight and inactive. Complications seen in both types are similar and usually related to duration of the disease. Both types can lead to development of:

- Coronary artery disease
- Stroke

- Diseases in the blood vessels of the extremities
- Nerve disorders
- Kidney problems

Diabetics who develop heart attacks or strokes are more likely to develop complications or die from these entities than are nondiabetics. Other complications, such as vision disturbances or complications of treatment (e.g., passing out from low blood sugar), can lead to falls, fractures, and automobile and work-related accidents.

Depression is found in up to 70 percent of patients with diabetic complications and significantly affects the course of the illness. Depressed diabetic patients are less in control of their diets, medications, and exercise programs.

Educating diabetics about the disease and the risk factors (diet, smoking, high blood pressure, high cholesterol, and lack of exercise) that speed its progression or complications can result in extensions of length and quality of life. Recent studies show that, in Type I diabetics, improved blood sugar control can delay significantly the onset and slow the progression of disease-related complications. Knowledgeable, up-to-date physicians interested in diabetes and skilled in teaching patients can be real assets to patients by overseeing good diabetic control and anticipating and helping prevent complications.

In the U.S., two-thirds of blindness before age 65 is due to diabetes. Because laser therapy has been shown to prevent progression of diabetic retinopathy, diabetic patients should be followed closely by ophthalmologists.

There has been debate for several decades about whether tight blood sugar control alters the course of complications in diabetes. Recently, the question has been answered for Type I diabetics who are early in the disease. Specifically, tight blood sugar control with home glucose monitoring and multiple insulin injections per day or insulin pump use has been shown to decrease the onset and progression of eye, kidney, and nerve complications. Tight blood sugar control has yet to be proven beneficial in avoiding complications for Type II diabetics, but a large study is underway to examine the issue.

Hypertension in both types is common and accelerates vascular disease. Control of blood pressure is, therefore, important in avoiding complications.

A blood pressure medication (angiotensin converting enzyme inhibitor) has been shown to slow progression of kidney disease in Type I patients.

Because diabetic patients already have vascular disease, smoking increases risks for cardiovascular complications; thus, smoking cessation is important for this population.

Recommendations
1. Become as knowledgeable as possible about your diabetes.
2. Enlist a physician who is interested in and knowledgeable about diabetes and its complications. You may wish to add an ophthalmologist and a dietitian to the team that will oversee your care.

3. Be in control of risk factors that could worsen control or increase complications of your diabetes; risk factors are cigarette smoking, high blood pressure, high cholesterol, obesity, and physical inactivity.

4. Keep your blood pressure below 130/85 mm Hg.

5. A good exercise program is extremely important.

6. If you have close relatives with diabetes, follow closely the large intervention trials that are aimed at preventing onset of the disease.

7. Watch the development of symptoms and signs that point to depression and share this information with your physician.

Further Reading

Verge CF and Eisenbarth GS: Strategies for preventing Type I diabetes mellitus. Western J Med;March 1996.

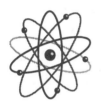

Bone Disease:
How to Avoid Brittle Bones and Fractures

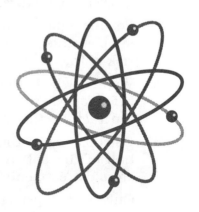

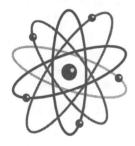

An archeologist is the best husband a woman can have; the older she gets, the more interested he is in her.

-Agatha Christie

Facts

1. By age 65, most women lose about 35 percent of their bone mass.

2. About 15 percent of all women eventually have hip fractures.

3. As many as 20 percent of patients die within a year of hip fracture.

4. Postmenopausal women who take estrogen supplements for five years can reduce their risk of fractures by about 50 percent.

5. Women whose mothers had hip fractures before age 80 are about twice as likely to have hip fractures themselves.

6. Osteoporosis is thought to occur in at least half of the patients who receive long-term steroid treatments.

7. Only a small percentage of patients who take long-term oral cortisone preparations ever receive treatment to prevent or treat osteoporosis.

Few people consider that bone-related problems are factors affecting longevity. Osteoporosis, a bone-thinning disease that leads to increased bone fragility and increased risk of fractures of the hip, spine, wrist, and ribs, is found in more than 25 million Americans, 80 percent of whom are women. As many as one of every two women and one in eight men who live past age 80 will have osteoporosis-related fractures. More than one million osteoporosis-related fractures are recorded each year in the U.S. About 70 percent of fractures in individuals ages 45 and older are of the types related to osteoporosis.

Osteoporosis is often thought of as a "silent" disease because bone loss occurs without symptoms and patients have no way of knowing their bones are becoming weak and fragile. The first awareness of osteoporosis may follow a fracture or collapsed vertebra occurring at the time of a fall, sudden strain, or bump.

Osteoporotic fracture rates increase significantly with age in both men and women; but at any age, the risk is twice as great in women as men. Elderly white women have about twice the incidence of fractures as African-American women.

Women can lose up to 20 percent of their bone mass in the five to seven years following menopause. This rapid bone loss makes them more susceptible to osteoporosis. Additionally, women have a greater propensity to falling and are more likely than men to survive to the age of vulnerability for falls and fractures.

Osteoporosis is responsible for more than 300,000 hip fractures each year in the U.S., about 840 fractures for every 100,000 persons over age 65. Hip fractures are not only associated with pain, discomfort, disability, and loss of independence but also have major effects on morbidity and mortality. Estimated expected survival is reduced 15 to 20 percent in the first year after a hip fracture. Though women have more hip fractures than men, the death rate for men within one year of hip fracture is 26 percent higher than for women. Adding to the problem is the fact that, of individuals living independently prior to a hip fracture, up to 25 percent remain in long-term care institutions a year later.

Causes of osteoporosis are not fully known, though it is known that certain people are more likely to develop the disease than others. Certain modifiable and unmodifiable risk factors are:

MODIFIABLE	UNMODIFIABLE
Low-calcium diet	Female sex
Anorexia nervosa or bulimia (forced vomiting)	Advanced age
Cigarette smoking	Caucasian or Asian race
Excessive alcohol intake	Small, thin frame
Inactive lifestyle	Family history
Immobilization	Early menopause
Malabsorption of calcium	Abnormal absence of menstrual periods
Low testosterone levels in men	
Endocrine disorders involving thyroid, adrenal, or pituitary glands	
Kidney and liver diseases and certain tumors	
Certain medications	

An important and frequently overlooked risk factor is the use of medications that can lead to bone damage. These medications include:

- Glucocorticoids (steroids)
- Excessive doses of thyroid hormone
- Seizure medications (e.g., Dilantin and barbiturates)
- Aluminum-containing antacids
- Heparin (long-term, high-dose use)
- Certain treatments for endometriosis
- Specialized medicines (e.g., methotrexate, cyclosporine A, cholestyramine)

Long-term oral cortisone preparations commonly used for arthritis, asthma, and chronic lung disease can often result in the development of osteoporosis and spinal and hip fractures. Only a small percentage of these drug patients are on programs to prevent complications, though several programs, e.g., hormone replacement therapy in postmenopausal women, appear promising. For those taking steroid medications, the American College of Rheumatology recommends that these patients take 1500 mg per day of calcium supplements, take at least 800 IU of vitamin D, and do weight bearing exercises for at least 30 to 60 minutes daily.

Because there is no real cure for osteoporosis, efforts to prevent its development are important. Treatments are available to help stop or slow further bone loss and resulting fractures, and estrogen can prevent bone loss in postmenopausal women. Certain other medications have specialized applications, and others are under investigation.

Approximately one-third of individuals ages 65 and older will fall each year. Falls can be due to:

- Various medications that cause:
  - Sedation
  - Lightheadedness
  - Dizziness
  - Loss of balance
  - Lowered blood pressure
- Combinations of medications that present special problems
- Loss of vision
- Loss of hearing
- Muscle weakness
- Loss of coordination
- Diseases that affect balance

Recommendations

1. Be aware of risk factors you may have for osteoporosis.

2. Ensure adequate calcium and vitamin D intake (see chart below).

3. Exercise.

4. Stop smoking.

5. Check with your doctor about medications you take that can cause osteoporosis, especially if you are in a high-risk category.

6. Understand the complications of falls and institute measures to avoid falling.

7. Make your home a safe environment with adequate lighting, hand rails, and attention to household hazards (e.g., loose carpeting, extension cords, toys).

8. Consider postmenopausal low-dose estrogen therapy.

OPTIMAL CALCIUM REQUIREMENTS

GROUP	OPTIMAL DAILY INTAKE (mg of calcium)*
Adolescents/Young Adults	
Ages 11 to 24	1,200 to 1,500
Men	
Ages 25 to 65	1,000
Over age 65	1,500
Women	
Ages 25 to 50	1,000
Over age 50 (postmenopausal):	
On estrogen	1,000
Not on estrogen	1,500
Over age 65	1,500
Pregnant and nursing	1,200 to 1,500

1 quart of milk has 1,000 mg of calcium
From Optimal Calcium Intake, NIH Consensus Statement, June 1994.

The average intake of calcium from our diets in the U.S. is probably less than 800 mg daily. When taking calcium supplements, it is best to take them with foods as absorption is then increased. Keeping single doses at 500 mg or less also helps absorption.

Vitamin D deficiency is associated with an increased risk of fractures. This is of special concern for the elderly because of:

- Insufficient dietary vitamin D intake
- Impaired renal synthesis of forms of vitamin D
- Inadequate sunlight exposure, common for many elderly

Providing elderly patients with 600 to 800 IU per day of vitamin D has been shown to reduce fracture risk.

Further Reading

Optimal Calcium Intake, NIH Censensus Statement. Vol 12, June, 1994.

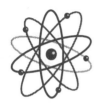

Dementia:
Not Inevitable in the Elderly

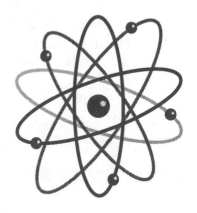

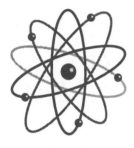

Happiness? That's nothing more than health and a poor memory.
                                           -Albert Schweitzer

Facts

1. At least one-third of individuals who reach age 85 have major impairments of memory and thinking, Alzheimer's disease most often being the cause.

2. Dementia affects up to 15 percent of people age 65 and older.

3. Dementia may be reversible in approximately 10 percent of patients.

4. Delirium and depression may be misdiagnosed as dementia.

5. Dementia occurs in up to 20 percent of patients with HIV infection.

6. A large variety and number of drugs lead to memory and/or thinking impairment.

Dementia is an acquired loss of memory and other mental skills that interfere with the performance of daily activities. Multiple areas of intellectual function are often affected, with areas of impairment including:

- Abstract thinking
- Language
- Judgment
- Perception
- Planning
- Problem-solving
- Memory

Important causes of dementia in older Americans include:

- Alzheimer's disease-50 to 85 percent
- Vascular disease-10 to 20 percent, which includes cerebrovascular phenomena such as:
  - Inflammation of blood vessels
  - Emboli or hemorrhages
  - Single or multiple brain infarctions
- Parkinson's Disease
- Brain tumors or trauma
- Infections, including:
  - HIV
  - Tuberculosis
  - Syphilis
  - Meningitis
  - Creutzfeldt-Jakob disease (caused by prions, a slow virus)
- Metabolic disorders, including:
  - Vitamin B_{12} deficiency
  - Hypothyroidism
- Alcohol abuse
- Poor nutrition
- Medications, either alone or in combination, such as those used for:

- Pain
- High blood pressure
- Sleep
- Sedation
- Treatment of psychiatric illnesses

Dementia is responsible for about 120,000 deaths annually, the mortality being strongly associated with its severity. Dementia patients are at increased risk for falls and automobile accidents; as many as 33 percent of demented persons who were still driving had motor vehicle crashes or moving violations within the previous six months, a fact suggesting potential for harm to patients, family members, and care-givers as well as to the public.

Dementia is commonly overlooked in its early stages, the time when reversible factors that cause or contribute to the disorder can be managed best. Finding and correcting underlying causes could result in improvement in some patients; these causes include:

- Depression
- Vitamin B_{12} deficiency
- Drug excess or toxicity
- Hypothyroidism
- Alcohol abuse
- Poor nutrition
- Space-occupying lesions (e.g., subdural hematoma)
- Normal pressure hydrocephalus

The number of demented patients who experience long-term improvement is relatively small. Some estimates suggest that 10 to 15 percent of dementia patients have a potentially reversible condition (e.g., drug intoxication, depression, or treatable glandular or nutritional disorder). Other studies have shown that about one-half of elderly dementia patients have at least one co-existing illness, the treatment of which could result in improvements for many patients.

Recommendations

1. If you have difficulty with memory, making judgements, or communicating with others, consult your physician or one specializing in dementia.

2. Be familiar with areas of impairment that suggest dementia.

3. When consulting a physician regarding dementia, bring a family member or close friend who is familiar with your day-to-day activities.

4. Check your family history for possible cases of dementia, realizing that diagnosis may have been missed or the symptoms attributed to aging.

5. Because a recent study suggested that estrogen replacement therapy may be associated with a lower risk for developing Alzheimer's disease, women should discuss this therapy with their physicians.

Further Reading

Fleming KC, Adams AC, Petersen RC: Dementia: Diagnosis and evaluation. Mayo Clinic Proceedings, November 1995.

Goldmacher DS and Whitehouse PJ: Evaluation of dementia. N Eng J Med August 1, 1996.

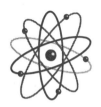

Infections/
HIV and the AIDS Epidemic

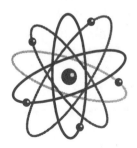

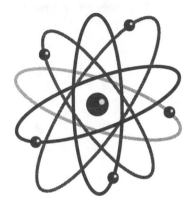

The biggest disease today is not leprosy or tuberculosis but rather the feeling of being unwanted.

-Mother Theresa

Facts

1. AIDS is the leading cause of death in the U.S. for those ages 25 to 44.

2. About 10 percent of AIDS cases in the U.S. occur in those ages 50 and older.

3. Estimates suggest that there are approximately one million asymptomatic carriers of the hepatitis B virus in the U.S.

4. Sixty to 80 percent of individuals who use illicit drugs intravenously have evidence of hepatitis B virus infection.

5. Severe pneumococcal bacterial infections result in death in 30 to 40 percent of elderly persons.

6. Influenza is the major cause of death due to infectious disease in the U.S., the last count suggesting 56,000 deaths per year.

At the turn of the century, the main causes of death in the U.S. were infectious diseases such as influenza, bacterial pneumonia, tuberculosis, and gastrointestinal infections. The development of vaccines and antibiotics, improved hygiene, regulations for food handling, and treated water supplies have led to major inroads in preventing and controlling these diseases; however, new and often difficult to treat infectious agents have proven to be major threats to public health. Viruses, especially HIV, hantavirus, and hepatitis viruses, recently have been of particular concern.

Today when considering infections that shorten life in significant numbers of people, HIV infection quickly comes to mind. AIDS, a term denoting the later stages of HIV infection with complications, has become the leading cause of death for people ages 25 to 44; recent data suggest that HIV/AIDS is the eighth leading cause of death in the U.S.

AIDS is not only a problem for young adults. About 10 percent of all cases diagnosed each year occur in both genders ages 50 and older. Increasing numbers from that group are from heterosexual transmission and probably are also related to this population's lack of knowledge about HIV infection, its characteristics, diagnosis, and transmission.

Current estimates suggest that 650,000 to 900,000 persons in the U.S. are infected with HIV, with approximately 40,000 new infections occurring each year. The vast majority of people infected with HIV will develop AIDS.

According to the Centers for Disease Control and Prevention, men who have sex with men and injection drug users account for more than 80 percent of AIDS cases. Most other cases result from:

- Transmission from mother to fetus
- Sexual partners of injection drug users
- Transfusion of infected blood or blood components

In theory, the virus can be spread by contact with an infected individual's feces, saliva, or urine, though such cases are rare. Individuals at high risk for HIV infection include:

- Men who have sex with men
- Injection drug users
- Sex partners of injection drug users
- Prostitutes and their sex partners
- Homosexual, bisexual, or heterosexual individuals who have had HIV-infected sex partners
- Those who have had blood product transfusions between 1978 and 1985
- Those having multiple sex partners, especially if engaging in unprotected sex (i.e., not using latex condoms)

Infections due to bacteria, viruses, and fungi are common throughout life and are found to varying degrees in different age groups. A modest number of infections in the U.S. are associated with a relatively high morbidity and mortality.

Pneumococcal bacterial disease can cause significant morbidity and mortality, especially in the elderly who, through aging, are thought to lose some immunologic functions, making them less able to contain infections. Pneumonia may be difficult to diagnose in the elderly, and some cases will be unresponsive or difficult to treat. In some cases, especially hospitalized patients, pneumonia can be prevented by careful feeding and attention to swallowing mechanisms of sick patients and, if possible, by avoiding tubes that assist with feeding or breathing in such patients.

A pneumococcal vaccine appears to be of value, with few adverse effects, for the elderly and especially institutionalized elderly, with the vaccine's protective effect appearing to last five to 10 years.

Influenza can cause significant morbidity and mortality during epidemics. The elderly are at increased risk for the major lethal complication of influenza (pneumonia). An effective influenza vaccine is available and can reduce mortality associated with influenza outbreaks. For the elderly or other individuals at high risk during a community outbreak, drugs (amantadine and rimantadine) can be used by those who have not already received the vaccine.

Tuberculosis (TB) rates are increasing in the U.S., especially among African-Americans, Hispanics, and Asians/Pacific Islanders. Up to 15 million persons in the U.S. are infected with the bacteria that causes TB, and foreign-born immigrants are a steady source of new cases. Individuals infected with HIV are more likely to develop active TB than others.

Major problems and increased mortality have been associated with the development of resistance to many of the standard drugs used to treat TB.

Skin tests and chest x-rays can help detect TB infection in exposed individuals who do not have symptoms. Such individuals include:

- Persons infected with HIV
- Persons in close contact with TB patients
- Health care workers
- Immigrants
- Residents of long-term care facilities
- Alcoholics
- Drug users

The finding of a newly positive TB skin test reaction is important because a drug, isoniazid, has proven effective in preventing the subsequent development of active TB in such individuals.

Viruses are also the cause of hepatitis B and C, both of which can cause severe liver damage in the form of cirrhosis and liver cancer. As many as 300,000 persons, mostly young adults, become infected with hepatitis B each year, the greatest risk coming from injecting illicit drugs but also commonly from sexual activity.

Health care workers are also at risk. A vaccine is available for hepatitis B but not C and should be given to those at increased risk, including:

- Health care workers
- Individuals with hemophilia
- Individuals living with infected persons
- Individuals at high risk
- Individuals traveling to parts of the world with a high prevalence of hepatitis B, particularly if engaged in risky behaviors (e.g., sexual activity)

Recommendations

1. Learn basic information about HIV infection and AIDS. Material is often provided by hospitals and public health departments.

2. If you are in a high-risk category for HIV infection (i.e., engaged in unprotected sex with a person of unknown HIV status), discuss this situation with your physician and obtain HIV testing.

3. Individuals with new or multiple sex partners should use latex condoms.

4. Seek monogamous sexual relationships with uninfected partners.

5. Patients ages 65 or older, ages 50 or older and living in institutional settings, or having problems such as diabetes, chronic heart or lung disease (emphysema), or chronic kidney problems should obtain pneumococcal vaccines. Patients who have had surgical removal of the spleen or have nonfunctional spleens (sickle cell disease) should obtain pneumococcal vaccines.

Further Reading

Guide to Clinical Preventive Services, Report of the U.S. Preventive Services Task Force, 2nd ed. Williams & Wilkins, 1996.

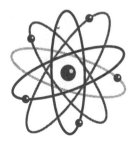

Sex: All You Want to Know

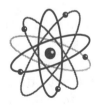

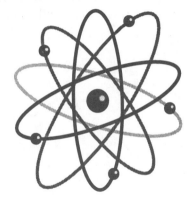

Really, sex and laughter do go very well together, and I wondered—and still do—which is the more important.

-Hermione Gingold

Facts

1. A high percentage of people experience sexual problems at some time in their lives, but many enjoy sex into their 80s.

2. Numerous medications can interfere with sexual functioning.

3. Between 10 and 20 million men in the U.S. are consistently unable to have an erection adequate for sexual intercourse.

4. About 85 percent of impotence is due to physical causes such as vascular disease, high blood pressure, diabetes, neurological problems, medications, smoking, or excessive alcohol. About 15 percent is caused by psychological problems.

To date, the authors have found no good studies to indicate that good sex extends life. However, few would deny that good sex throughout life makes life more enjoyable. Good or bad sex is somewhat difficult to define. Probably easiest is to say that the sexual experience depends on whatever the involved couple mutually finds satisfying or unsatisfying.

For satisfying sexual function to occur, there must be a complex interaction of psychological, nervous, vascular, and endocrine systems. Problems involving one of more of those systems interfere with normal sexual function, and the resulting sexual dysfunction can lead to interpersonal problems for the couple, which can worsen the sexual difficulties.

Sexual dysfunction, as manifest by changes in sexual desire and ability, can be the manifestation of:

- An underlying emotional or psychiatric disorder
- Anxiety
- Stress
- Depression
- Schizophrenia
- Dementia

Professional help from physicians or designated specialists may be needed in many cases.

Sexual dysfunction may also be an early manifestation of an illness that, in one way or another, interferes with interactions of the nervous, vascular, and endocrine systems. Impotence, the inability to achieve an erection adequate for sexual intercourse, is a distressing problem for men that can be caused by a variety of illnesses; recognized disorders include:

- ○ Conditions involving the brain and spinal cord, including:
    - ○ Parkinson's disease
    - ○ Multiple Sclerosis
    - ○ Strokes
    - ○ Herniated discs
- ○ Certain blood vessel disorders
- ○ Hypertension
- ○ Coronary artery disease
- ○ Endocrine disorders, including:
    - ○ Diabetes mellitus
    - ○ Thyroid disorders

Low levels of the male hormone testosterone are responsible for only a small percentage of impotence cases.

Unfortunately, correction or control of illnesses may not always eliminate sexual dysfunction. However, if the dysfunction is caused by a medication, the problem can often be resolved.

Drugs that interfere with sexual function include:

- ○ High blood pressure medications, including:
    - ○ Diuretics (thiazides, spironolactone)
    - ○ Catapres
    - ○ Aldomet
    - ○ Beta-blockers
    - ○ Hydralazine
    - ○ Reserpine
    - ○ Guanethidine
    - ○ Prazosin
    - ○ Estrogen

- Recreational, abused, or illicit drugs, including:
  - Alcohol
  - Tobacco
  - Cocaine
  - Heroin
  - Opiates
- Antidepressant medications, including:
  - Tricylics (e.g., Elavil)
  - Monoamine oxidase inhibitors
  - Trazodone
  - Serotonin re-uptake inhibitors (e.g. Prozac)
- Drugs that act on the central nervous system, including:
  - Phenytoin (Dilantin)
  - Barbiturates
  - Phenothiazines
- Others, including:
  - Antihistamines/decongestants
  - Cimetidine
  - Cancer chemotherapeutic agents
  - Clofibrate
  - Tranquilizers
  - Digoxin
  - Estrogen

A relatively common recent problem is the use/abuse of high doses of anabolic steroids by recreational body builders. Use of these agents can be associated with a wide range of serious complications.

The good news for men with impotence is that most can be helped. Aphrodisiacs do not work; nor do such popular items as ginseng, rhinoceros horn, melatonin, or various other herbs. Items that do work are:

○ Vacuum devices
○ A medication that is easily injected into the penis
○ A new urethral suppository that appears effective
○ Various penis-like implants that are placed surgically

Of interest is the fact that, because erectile dysfunction is commonly associated with cardiovascular disease, good control of cardiovascular risk factors should be good for sexual performance; especially important are:

○ Exercise
○ Diet
○ Alcohol restriction
○ Not smoking

A study at the University of South Carolina School of Medicine found that men whose total cholesterol was greater than 240 mg/dl were almost twice as likely to become impotent as those whose cholesterol was below 180 mg/dl. Studies at Duke University also suggest that cholesterol-blocked vessels may slow the flow of blood to the penis, which contributes to impotence.

A common source of anxiety related to sexual activity occurs after a heart attack or coronary bypass surgery. The concern is that sexual intercourse may trigger another heart attack. However, studies suggest that heart attack patients who are otherwise doing well have little, if any, risk from sexual intercourse and should be able to resume sexual activity during the second week after hospital discharge. One recognized source of increased risk, however, is having sex with a person other than the usual partner.

It has been suggested that sexual intercourse as an exercise might be the equivalent of climbing about 20 stairs. If this is true, it is better understood why sexual activity as an exercise factor, or cholesterol burner, does not contribute to life extension. On the other hand, a happy wife is more likely to see that her husband gets his five servings of fruits and vegetables daily, avoids depression, takes his medications, and visits his doctor.

Recommendations

1. If you experience sexual dysfunction problems, do not hesitate to seek professional help.

2. Communicate to your partner the sexual feelings and behaviors in which you would like to engage.

3. Remember that certain diseases and various drugs can cause sexual dysfunction.

4. Most couples eventually experience some form of sexual problems that can be satisfactorily resolved by knowledgeable, caring physicians.

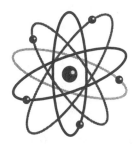

Injuries/Accidents/ Domestic Violence

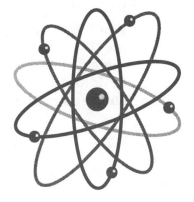

With a good heredity, nature deals you a fine hand at cards; and with good environment, you learn to play the hand well.

-Walter C. Alvarez, M.D.

Facts

1. Injury is the third leading cause of death in the U.S.

2. Motor vehicle crash-related injuries are the eighth leading cause of death in the U.S.

3. Falls are the second leading cause of unintentional injury death in the U.S.

4. Smoking materials have been implicated in up to 33 percent of residential-fire deaths among the elderly.

5. Increased use of automobile safety restraints contributed to a 32-percent decline in the death rate from car crashes.

6. Domestic violence is the leading cause of injury to women in the U.S., with an estimated 4,000 women killed each year. Battering accounts for about one-half of all serious injuries in women presenting to emergency departments.

7. When compared with nonsmokers, smokers are 1.5 times more likely to have a motor vehicle crash, 1.4 to 2.5 times more likely to be injured at work, and twice as likely to suffer other unintentional injuries.

Injury is an important cause of death in the U.S., accounting each year for about 4.3 million potential years of life lost prematurely before age 70. Injuries are not necessarily accidents, i.e., those that occur by chance and are unavoidable because they usually can be attributed to preventable behavioral and environmental factors. Important causes of injuries include:

- Motor vehicle crashes
- Burns
- Drowning
- Poisoning
- Falls

Injuries commonly occur in the workplace. In the U.S., 17 work-related fatalities occur each day; their leading causes are:

- Motor vehicles - 23 percent
- Machines - 13 percent
- Homicides - 12 percent
- Falls - 10 percent
- Electrocutions - 7 percent
- Strikes by falling objects - 7 percent
- All others - 28 percent

(From *For a Healthy Nation*, U.S. Department of Health and Human Services, Public Health Service.)

Motor vehicle crash-related injuries are important causes of death. Motor vehicle fatality rates are highest for the young and elderly. Drivers ages 70 and older have more fatalities than middle-aged drivers, related to:

- Loss of vision
- Loss of hearing
- Dulled reaction times

Dementia particularly impairs driving ability, as do alcohol and sleep disorders.

All drivers should recognize the value of:
- Seat belts
- Helmets (bicycle or motorcycle)
- Air bags
- Periodic vision and hearing exams
- Driving free of the influence of:
  - Alcohol
  - Illicit drugs
  - Certain over-the-counter medications
  - Certain prescription medications

Many medications have mind-altering effects. About one-third of drivers killed in crashes are intoxicated by alcohol. Drugs such as marijuana, cocaine, and tranquilizers are also important contributors to lethal crashes.

Wearing a seat belt can increase the survival rate of car crash passengers by one-half. Those thrown from vehicles are 24 to 40 times more likely to be killed. Your physician may comment and advise you on the habits, physical or mental deficiencies, or prescribed medications that can hamper your ability to drive or operate machines that require significant skill and attention.

At least one-third of older adults fall each year in the U.S., resulting in about 12,000 deaths. Falls by elderly people lead to injuries, such as hip fractures, which in turn result in death 10 to 20 percent of the time.

Some environmental risk factors can be corrected to help prevent falls; risk factors include:

- Pavement irregularities
- Slippery floors
- Poor lighting
- Poor-fitting or inadequate shoe size

Helping to protect against falls, especially for the elderly, are:

- Exercise programs
- Gait retraining
- Gait aids
- Adequate vision correction
- Recognition of medication side effects

Burn injuries, most commonly flame and scald injuries, have the highest mortality for those ages 60 and older. Cigarette smoking is an important cause of fire and burn injury deaths and is associated with about 25 percent of residential fires. Homes often do not have smoke detectors, and sometimes elderly patients may not hear or be able to respond to alarms. Avoiding smoking, especially in bed, and attention to the temperatures of tap water, food, and drinks can greatly reduce the incidence of fire and burn injuries.

Unintentional poisonings lead to a significant number of deaths among adults, the highest incidence being in young adult men. Most of these deaths are related to overdose of alcohol or drugs such as heroin and cocaine. Elderly patients with arthritis or other painful problems may excessively use aspirin and/or other pain relievers that can lead to:

- Gastrointestinal bleeding
- Confusion
- Kidney failure
- Pulmonary edema

In the U.S. each year, four to eight million women, from all cultural and socioeconomic groups, suffer physical abuse inflicted by their spouses or partners. Adult women are more likely to be sexually assaulted, beaten, and killed in their own homes at the hands of their male partners than any place else or by anyone else in society.

Estimates also suggest that up to two million cases of elder abuse occur annually in the U.S. This is of particular concern as the population ages. The mistreatment of the elderly may be even more difficult to identify because of:

- The relative isolation of this group
- The tendency not to report this form of abuse
- The subtle forms that this abuse can take so that it is often undetected

Help for such victims involves community efforts that include individuals, agencies, health care facilities, and law enforcement organizations who are motivated to work together for the reduction and prevention of violence. Victims should understand that they can initiate help simply by calling 911. Getting to a hospital emergency room will also initiate desired assistance.

Recommendations

1. If you have been drinking alcoholic or using mind-altering drugs, do not drive or operate potentially dangerous machinery.

2. If you have difficulty walking or have frequent falls, inform your physician, who will look for and work to correct reversible causes.

3. Do not smoke, especially in bed.

4. Be sure to have periodic vision and hearing tests.

5. Always wear a seat belt or helmet (motorcycle or bicycle).

6. Recognize that medicines you take may have potential mind-altering effects.

7. Learn what facilities your community has for aiding victims of domestic violence.

Further Reading

Scheitel SM, Fleming KC, Chutha DS, Evans JM: Geriatric Health Maintenance, Mayo Clinic Proceedings, March 1966.

Guide to Clinical Preventive Services, Report of the U.S. Preventive Services Task Force, 2nd ed. Williams & Wilkins, 1996.

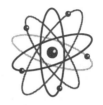

The Bad (Polypharmacy) and the Ugly (Cocaine)

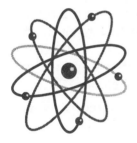

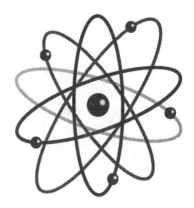

There are some remedies worse than the disease.

-Pubblius Syrus

Facts

1. Elderly Americans (ages 65 and over) account for the purchase of 30 percent of all prescription drugs and 40 percent of over-the-counter drugs.

2. Age-related changes in elderly patients allow drugs to maintain their effects longer, have unusual or unexpected actions, and cause more adverse reactions with serious or potentially life-threatening outcomes.

3. The average nursing home patient receives four to seven different medications daily.

4. Cocaine-related injuries are a major cause of death among young adults in areas such as New York City.

5. A heart attack is the most commonly reported cardiac complication of cocaine abuse.

6. Chest pain is the most common cocaine-related medical problem, resulting in the evaluation of more than 64,000 patients annually for possible coronary artery problems.

During the last 30 years, the number of FDA-approved drugs available for the treatment of diseases and their medical complications has increased from 650 to more than 9,500, and of those there are approximately 1,000 generic compounds. The shear volume of drugs makes it impossible, without the aid of sophisticated computer systems, for physicians to master knowledge of the complex actions of specific drugs, their complications, their interactions with other drugs, and their altered activities in various disease states. Fortunately, recent developments have made more drug information available so that physicians may keep abreast of the latest findings.

Polypharmacy

The seriousness of problems related to adverse drug events is apparent, considering that:

- Prescription-related drug problems result in about 119,000 annual U.S. deaths

- Twenty-eight percent of hospitalized patients experience adverse drug events annually, translating to 8.8 million hospitalizations each year

- Tens of thousands of fatalities in hospitalized patients in the U.S. occur annually due to drugs

- One in four people ages 65 and older receive at least one of 20 drugs that are potentially inappropriate for elderly patients

- Thirty percent of elderly patients use eight or more prescription drugs daily, and the elderly population takes an average of 18 prescription drugs per year

- It is estimated that 10 to 30 percent of hospital admissions among the elderly are related to drug problems such as:
  - Inappropriate drug prescribing
  - Noncompliance
  - Adverse drug events

Elderly people are especially prone to adverse drug events because of their intake of multiple medications and their incidence of multiple chronic diseases. This problem is of particular concern because the elderly population is expected to increase from 31 million in 1989 to 52 million in the year 2020.

Cocaine

In a particular year, more than four million Americans use cocaine, with about one-third of those using cocaine monthly. Though figures are difficult to determine, it has been estimated that more than 20 million Americans have tried cocaine at least once.

Cocaine can cause problems no matter what the route of administration—intranasal, smoking, or intravenous injection. Cocaine can be directly related to a variety of problems, including:
- Heart attacks
- Seizures
- Respiratory distress
- Mental problems

Indirectly, it can be associated with:
- Homicides
- Suicides
- Motor vehicle accidents

Heart attacks are the most commonly reported cardiac complication of cocaine use. Even small amounts of the drug can trigger such an event, even in the first-time user. Heart attacks can occur shortly after use or on the following day and can occur in a young person with normal coronary arteries, suggesting the occurrence of spasm and occlusion of a coronary artery.

Cocaine can also cause sudden death by other mechanisms, such as:

- Heart rhythm disturbances
- Strokes
- Sudden major increases in blood pressure

Besides the drug itself, certain adulterants found in street cocaine can present major problems.

Recommendations

1. At least once a year, bag all your pills, take them to your doctor, and ask if you still need them and if there are any you can do without.

2. Remember that a medication (or combination of medications) you take could explain a worsening of your condition, new symptoms, or even a new illness.

3. Learn as much as you can about your medications. Elderly patients should ask for help (from family, friends, caregivers, etc.) with this sometimes burdensome task.

4. NEVER, EVER, USE ANY FORM OF COCAINE.

5. If already dependent on cocaine, seek the assistance of your physician or a substance-abuse specialist.

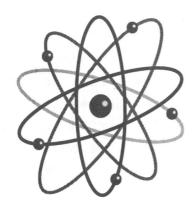

Smoking:
Enormous Complications of
Addiction and Powerful
Benefits from Quitting

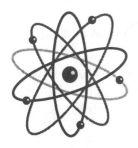

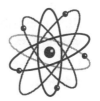

Tobacco drieth the brain, dimmeth the sight, vitiateth the smell, hurteth the stomach, destroyeth the concoction, disturbeth the humors and spirits, corrupteth the breath, induceth a trembling of the limbs, exiccateth the windpipe, lungs and liver, annoyeth the milt, scorcheth the heart, and causeth the blood to be adjusted.

- Tobias Venner

Facts

1. An average smoker dies eight years earlier than a nonsmoker.

2. Studies suggest that 30 to 40 percent of the half million yearly U.S. deaths from coronary heart disease are due to smoking.

3. Smoking only one to four cigarettes a day can more than double the risk of death from coronary artery disease.

4. Smoking is the cause of 30 percent of all deaths from cancer.

5. Nonsmokers living with smokers have a 30-percent higher risk of dying from heart disease than do nonsmokers without such exposure.

6. Cigarette smoking is the number one preventable cause of premature death in the U.S.

7. A 40-year study of British physicians has predicted that about half of all regular smokers will eventually die as a result of cigarette use.

Smoking and other tobacco use has been chosen as the first risk factor discussed in this book because it best exemplifies the concept that is hoped to be relayed to readers—that one's life can be extended significantly by certain reasonable actions. The best and most recent data indicate that smoking-related illnesses account for nearly one in five deaths and more than one-fourth of all deaths among those ages 35 to 64. It has been estimated that during the 1990s in developed countries, tobacco use will cause about 30 percent of all deaths among this age group, making smoking the largest single cause of premature death in the developed world.

In the U.S., the best recent estimate, when those who die from passive smoking (the breathing of sidestream smoke emitted from burning tobacco) are included, is that tobacco kills about 480,000 people each year and causes about 180,000 deaths from cardiovascular disease (coronary artery disease and stroke).

Heart disease, not cancer, is the main disease caused by smoking. Though heavy smoking for long periods is generally recognized as a problem, smokers tend to ignore studies that show that lesser exposures can also be lethal. In one major study of nurses, it was found that those nurses who smoked one to four cigarettes daily had a 2.5-fold increased risk of fatal coronary artery disease and nonfatal heart attacks when compared to nonsmoking nurses. Some individuals are so sensitive to tobacco smoke that the mere entrance into a smoke-filled room can cause their coronary arteries to go into spasm, occlude blood flow, and cause chest pain and possible damage to the heart muscle.

Cigarette smoking is responsible for 30 percent of all deaths from cancer and represents the most important preventable cause of cancer in the U.S. Besides causing 85 percent of lung cancer, smoking is also associated with cancers of the:

o   Mouth
o   Throat
o   Larynx
o   Esophagus
o   Stomach
o   Pancreas
o   Cervix
o   Kidney
o   Ureter
o   Bladder
o   Colon

As occurs with heart disease, cancer, in certain unfortunate individuals, can be caused by short periods of exposure to relatively small numbers of cigarettes. Passive smoking, such as exposure to parents' smoke during childhood and adolescence as well as exposure from living with a spouse who smokes or working with fellow employees who smoke, is also a recognized cause of lung and other cancers. Cigarette smoking is also the leading cause of lung illness and death in the U.S., causing more than 84,000 deaths from such problems as:

o   Emphysema
o   Pneumonia
o   Bronchitis

Problems related to use of tobacco products are present at each and every age. An article in *Time* magazine reported that even three insurance firms owned by tobacco companies charge smokers nearly double for term life insurance because smokers are about twice as likely to die at a given age.

The hazards of smoking extend well into later life. Among those over age 65, the rates of total mortality among current smokers were twice that of those who never smoked. Oral cancers in men who use smokeless tobacco (snuff, chewing tobacco), typically occur in the over age 65 group, though it can be seen much earlier.

The recent resurgence of cigar smoking overlooks the fact that there is no safe form of tobacco, just as there is no safe period of time for tobacco use. Estimates of deaths from pipe and cigar smoking just prior to the recent increase in cigar sales were 14,000 yearly in the U.S. Surely this number will increase if the trend continues.

Many smokers are switching to lower tar and nicotine cigarette brands rather than quitting, in the misguided belief that they can smoke more safely. A wealth of scientific evidence contradicts this strategy, however, because smokers inhale these low-yield cigarettes more deeply and smoke more of them to obtain the same nicotine kick.

Those fortunate enough to escape death from tobacco toxin exposure can still find themselves compromised in later life by damaged hearts or emphysematous lungs. These and other consequences of tobacco-related injuries can make afflicted individuals more at risk for other illnesses (pneumonia, stroke) common to later life.

Much still can be gained by those who, after any period of using any quantity or variety of tobacco (cigarettes, cigars, pipes, snuff, or chewing tobacco) at any age, are able to kick the habit, provided the lethal condition has not yet become manifest:

- After about a year, mortality from heart disease drops halfway back to that of nonsmokers and after five years to the rate equal to nonsmokers
- Risk of lung cancer is cut in half in five years and after 10 years drops to the rate of nonsmokers
- Lifelong smokers who quit at age 50 double their chances of living to age 65

Smokers who die between ages 35 and 64 lose 23 years of life compared to age-matched nonsmokers.

Today smokers are quitting in large numbers with the help of sympathetic physicians and through the use of:

- Nicotine patches and gums (which can be purchased over-the-counter)
- Behavior modification programs
- Effective medicines for associated anxiety
- The almost daily reports in the media regarding the dangers of tobacco
- Acknowledgements of subversive activities of the tobacco industry

Recommendations

1. If you are a smoker, quit. If you chew tobacco, stop.

2. If you live with a smoker, discuss your concerns for your health with him/her and review data together. Your goal should be that smokers not smoke in your presence or in rooms that you

frequent or, if possible, anywhere in your house. Tobacco toxins have tremendous capabilities of moving from room to room and from one floor to another.

3. If you are exposed to passive smoke at work, discuss your concerns with fellow employees or your boss. It may be necessary to change jobs. Your personal physician may be able to document your distress or risks from such exposure. Studies have shown added risk for those exposed to passive smoking both at home and at work.

4. For help quitting smoking, seek the assistance of your physician or a physician skilled in smoking cessation programs. Because smokers have more depression, physicians may detect and treat this in the process of supporting their patients' tobacco cessation programs.

5. Tips for individuals who require extra assistance in quitting are listed below.

Further Reading

Bartecchi CE, MacKenzie TD, Schrier RW: The human cost of tobacco use. New Eng J Med March 31 and April 7, 1994.

Bartecchi CE, MacKenzie TD, Schrier RW: The global tobacco epidemic. Sci Am May 1995.

Clearing the air: How to quit smoking and quit for keeps. Prepared by the Office of Cancer Communications, National Cancer Institute. NIH Publication No. 89-1647, February 1989.

Smoking facts and tips for quitting. National Institutes of Health, National Cancer Institute. NIH Publication No. 93-3405, September 1993.

Tips to Help You Stop Smoking

Patients should realize that approximately 40 million Americans have quit smoking and that about 95 percent of these stopped on their own without any formal cessation program. Quitting rates are about twice as high for those who quit on their own as for those who participate in formal smoking cessation programs.

Of the various strategies for quitting, those who do so "cold turkey" are more likely to remain abstinent. Ongoing encouragement and assistance from physicians has also been cited by successful quitters as important in their decisions to quit and in preventing relapses.

Those who want to quit smoking should realize that some short-term discomforts/withdrawal symptoms will occur; these include:

- Dry mouth
- Sore throat
- Sore gums
- Sore tongue
- Headache
- Trouble sleeping
- Fatigue
- Hunger
- Tenseness
- Irritability
- Coughing

These symptoms peak within a few days but usually last only a week or two. Relapses can occur in the first week after quitting and even for months afterwards, and these can be particularly hard times. Slips may occur, especially during periods of emotional turmoil, but should not be equated with total failure. It is important to keep trying. Many successful quitters failed repeatedly before they were finally able to quit.

A great deal of experience with smokers and their efforts to quit has led organizations such as the National Institutes of Health, the National Cancer Institute, and the American Heart Association to recommend the following tips to help smokers in their efforts to quit.

GETTING READY TO QUIT
1. Select a target date for quitting, possibly a special day, such as a birthday, anniversary, or holiday.

2. Decide positively that you want to quit. Try to avoid negative thoughts about how difficult it might be.

3. List all the reasons why you want to quit. Write them down and carry them with you. Read them whenever you are tempted to smoke.

4. Notice when and why you smoke. Try to find the things in your daily life that you often do while smoking, such as drinking your morning cup of coffee or talking on the telephone.

5. Change your smoking routines. Keep your cigarettes in a different place, make them difficult to find. Smoke with your other hand.

6. Smoke only in certain places, such as outdoors, or in places that are uncomfortable.

7. Begin to condition yourself physically. Start a modest exercise program, drink more fluids, get plenty of rest, and avoid fatigue.

8. Choose your environment. Spend more and more time in places where smoking is not allowed.

9. Ask your spouse or a friend to quit with you. Share your feelings and offer mutual support.

10. Switch to a brand of cigarettes you find distasteful.

11. Collect all your cigarette butts in one large glass container to remind yourself of the filth that smoking represents. Don't empty your ashtrays. This will remind you how many cigarettes you smoke each day.

12. Smoke only those cigarettes you really want. Catch yourself before you light up a cigarette out of pure habit.

13. Think of quitting in terms of one day at a time.

THE DAY YOU QUIT

1. Throw away all your cigarettes and matches. Put away your lighters and ashtrays.

2. Change your morning routine. When you eat breakfast, sit at a different place at the table. Stay busy, exercise, go to the movies.

3. When you get the urge to smoke, do something else instead. Try to replace the urge by chewing sugarless gum or mints. Snack on celery or carrots.

4. Remind family and friends that this is your quit date and ask for their help over the next couple of weeks.

5. Carry other things to put in your mouth, such as gum, hard candy, or a toothpick.

6. Spend this day and following days with non-smokers and in places where smoking is not allowed.

7. Drink large quantities of water and fruit juices (avoid caffeine beverages).

8. Avoid alcohol, coffee, or other beverages that you associate with cigarette smoking.

9. If you miss the sensation of having a cigarette in your hand, play with something else, such as a pencil, paper clip, or marble.

10. Visit your dentist and have your teeth cleaned to get rid of tobacco stains.

11. Reward yourself at the end of the day. Estimate the amount of money you saved and buy yourself a treat, such as a movie or a book, and enjoy your favorite meal.

12. Limit your socializing to healthful, outdoor activities and sports in situations in which it would be difficult to smoke.

13. Don't allow yourself to think that "one cigarette won't hurt." It will!

STAYING OFF CIGARETTES

1. Don't worry if you are sleepier or more short-tempered than usual. These feelings will pass.

2. Begin to increase your exercise program.

3. Review in your mind the positive things about quitting, such as how much you like yourself as a nonsmoker and the health benefits to you and your family. A positive attitude can help through rough times.

4. When you feel tense, try to keep busy. Think about ways to solve the problem; tell yourself smoking won't make it any better; and do something else.

5. Eat regular meals. Feeling hungry is sometimes mistaken for the desire to smoke.

6. Start a money jar with the money you save by not buying cigarettes.

7. Let others know you quit smoking. Most people will support you.

8. If you slip and smoke, don't be discouraged. Many former smokers tried to stop several times before they finally succeeded. Quit again.

9. Watch your food and calorie intake so as not to gain weight during this period. Count calories if necessary. Increased exercise can help burn calories.

10. Follow-up visits with your physician, usually at the end of the second week, may prove helpful. Further help in the form of extra motivation, advice, and/or nicotine gum or patches might be suggested or instituted.

11. Watch out for triggers that are commonly recognized as stimulating a sudden, intense urge to smoke, such as:
   ○ Working under pressure
   ○ Feeling blue
   ○ Talking on the telephone
   ○ Having a drink
   ○ Watching television
   ○ Driving your car
   ○ Finishing a meal
   ○ Playing cards
   ○ Drinking coffee
   ○ Watching someone else smoke

12. When possible, support new taxes that raise the price of cigarettes, making the smoking habit even more painful.

13. Periodically, write down new reasons why you're happy you quit and post these where you'll be sure to see them.

This extensive, though not exhaustive list is not meant to be burdensome to the potential quitter. The authors recommend reviewing the list and selecting those items you can implement successfully, realizing that all have value and have proven effective for some individuals.

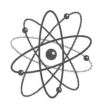

Good and Bad Cholesterol: Implications for Cardiovascular Disease

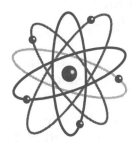

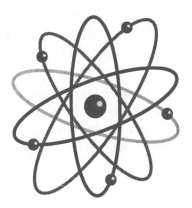

As I see it, every day you do one of two things: build health or produce disease in yourself.

-Adelle Davis

Facts

1. At any cholesterol level, a 10-percent increase in serum cholesterol is associated with a 20-percent or greater increased risk of coronary artery disease.

2. A 10-percent reduction in serum cholesterol could result in as much as a 10-percent reduction in death from coronary artery disease.

3. About 40 million Americans are thought to have cholesterol levels high enough to require medical attention.

4. Studies suggest that only 45 to 65 percent of patients with high cholesterol had evidence of treatment.

5. Newer drugs that have been shown to lower cholesterol in patients with cardiovascular diseases also have been shown to prolong life significantly.

6. These newer drugs, often called "statins", not only have the ability to decrease the risk of the first or subsequent heart attack or stroke but also have the capacity to prevent such problems from occurring at all.

Cholesterol is a soft, waxy, fat-like substance that is produced only by animals, is normally found throughout the body, and is necessary for healthy body function. The substance becomes a problem when too much is present and is deposited in the wrong places, such as in the coronary arteries or arteries leading to the brain or blood vessels in the legs.

Cholesterol travels throughout the body in the blood stream packaged in units called lipoproteins:

- Low-density lipoprotein (LDL), also known as bad cholesterol, is the main cholesterol-carrying compound in the blood. It plays an important role in plaque formation within arteries

- High-density lipoprotein (HDL), also known as good cholesterol, helps remove cholesterol from arteries and transports it to the liver for clearance from the bloodstream

- Very-low-density lipoprotein (VLDL) transports triglycerides to the tissues where they are broken down and used for energy or are stored. Triglyceride formation is increased when excess calories are present

Some people inherit a disorder that results in high cholesterol levels and early-onset, severe coronary artery disease. Others have cholesterol problems due to lifestyle choices such as diet, inactivity, or smoking. Some have combinations of these entities.

Levels of fats in the blood can be determined by direct measurements or formulas. Total cholesterol, the most common test, is made up of LDL, HDL, and other blood lipid particles. Some helpful numbers to remember for individuals without known heart disease are:

Cholesterol Type (mg/dl)	Desirable	Borderline	Undesirable
Total Cholesterol	<200	200-239	>240
HDL Cholesterol	>45	35-44	<35
LDL Cholesterol	<130	130-160	>160
Triglycerides	<200	200-400	>400

Even stricter goals are set for those with known heart disease. A recent study of patients who had heart attacks suggests there is considerable benefit derived from treatment with lipid-lowering drugs, even if LDL cholesterol is not above 130. Such treatment could involve as many as four million people. Some specialists even recommend using a "statin" drug to treat all coronary artery disease patients with LDL cholesterol levels above 100 unless such patients have contraindications to taking such drugs.

At present there is much controversy about who should be screened for high cholesterol. Physicians will inform their patients about which tests are needed, when they are needed, and how patients should prepare for them. Certainly those at risk for coronary artery disease, those who have had heart attacks, and middle-aged men with cardiac risk factors are in need of screening studies. Family or personal histories of cholesterol or vascular problems (strokes) suggest benefit from screening. Abnormal cholesterol studies are of less value in persons ages 70 and older unless they are known to have coronary artery disease.

Finding elevated total blood cholesterol in young or middle-aged individuals suggests the need to measure the other lipoprotein levels. For those at risk, the higher the total cholesterol level, the greater the risk of cardiovascular disease. This risk is further increased if LDL is high and HDL is low, a particularly bad combination. Under any circumstances, however, high LDL is undesirable because it causes atherosclerosis. However, low HDL by itself is also of concern.

Triglyceride levels are not as helpful as measurements of LDL and HDL. For age groups at risk for coronary artery disease, the lower the LDL and higher the HDL, the less likely heart attacks will occur. Abnormal cholesterol tests when combined with other risk factors increase significantly the risks of developing cardiovascular disease. Other risk factors are:

- High blood pressure
- Diabetes
- Age
- Male gender
- Smoking
- Obesity
- Family history
- Lack of exercise
- Lower socioeconomic status

The presence of several risk factors further magnifies the problem in such individuals. Those who are placed in the high-risk group due to the combination of cholesterol tests and risk factors should seek their physicians' help to outline programs of cholesterol control and risk factor reduction. It is suggested that for each one-percent reduction in blood cholesterol, there may be a two-percent reduction in heart attack risk.

Little can be said about triglycerides, mainly because the data are not complete about this fat. It is known that triglycerides can be elevated in diabetes and thyroid, liver, and kidney diseases. Certain drugs, even oral estrogens in some women, and alcohol in excess can also raise triglyceride levels.

High triglyceride levels on their own or especially in combination with other cholesterol problems appear to be associated with coronary artery disease, and very high triglyceride levels can precipitate bouts of pancreatitis. In any case, elevated triglycerides should indicate:

- Weight loss for obese patients
- Dietary manipulation
- Exercise
- Reduction of alcohol intake

Some individuals may require drug treatment.

Good programs are available for control of abnormal cholesterol levels; however, diet and exercise should form the basis of any program. Weight loss for obese patients is definitely helpful, and increasing fiber intake can lower cholesterol levels. For postmenopausal women, adding estrogen can lower cholesterol levels.

For some patients with high cholesterol, especially those with existing heart disease, cholesterol-lowering drugs may be needed, some of which have proven efficacy in preventing heart attacks and lowering death rates.

Best of all, improvements in coronary arteries due to cholesterol reduction can occur within months of initiating treatment. Presently available drugs appear to be able to stabilize lesions in coronary arteries and thus prevent rupture of obstructing plaque, which can lead to occlusion of coronary vessels and heart attack. Effective drug programs require close cooperation between patients and physicians, because these drugs can have serious side effects.

Lipid-lowering drug programs are usually long-term efforts. Unfortunately, about 50 percent of patients on drug programs discontinue drug therapy on their own within one year. Only about 25 percent of patients continue drug therapy through the end of the second year.

Recommendations
1. Know your cholesterol levels.
2. Know the risk factors you have and eliminate or control as many as possible.
3. Follow a regular exercise program.
4. Eat at least five servings of fruits and vegetables daily.
5. Become familiar with the American Heart Association prudent diet.
6. Middle-aged men with high cholesterol and/or other risk factors may consider having one to two alcoholic drinks daily. Alcohol intake in excess of one to two drinks per day is <u>not</u> recommended.
7. If a low-cholesterol, low-fat diet does not control your lipid problem, you may be a candidate for cholesterol-lowering drugs to be used along with your diet.

8. Follow closely the National Cholesterol Education Program (NCEP) guidelines for LDL cholesterol goals as summarized below:

FOR INDIVIDUALS WITH:	LDL CHOLESTEROL GOAL:
Definite coronary heart disease (CHD) or other atherosclerotic disease	≤100 mg/dL
No CHD but with two or more other CHD risk factors**	<130 mg/dL
No CHD and with fewer than two other CHD risk factors**	<160 mg/dL

**NCEP Risk Factors:

Age: ≥45 years in men and ≥55 years in women or women with premature menopause not using estrogen replacement therapy

Family history of premature CHD

Current cigarette smoking

Hypertension (BP ≥140/90 mm Hg) or taking antihypertensive medication

Diabetes mellitus

Low HDL cholesterol (<35 mg/dL) or subtract one risk factor if HDL cholesterol is ≥60 mg/dL

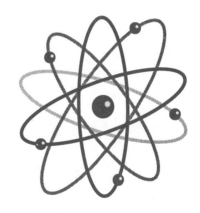

Obesity:
Benefits of and Approaches to
Weight Loss

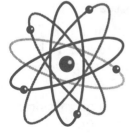

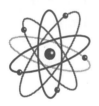

More die in the United States of too much food than of too little.

-John Kenneth Galbraith

Facts

1. One-third of adults in the U.S. are overweight.

2. Individuals who are 20 percent or more over ideal body weight are at higher risk of developing coronary artery disease.

3. Individuals who are 40 percent or more over ideal body weight are at much higher risk of cancers of the colon, prostate, breast, gallbladder, ovary, uterus, and cervix.

4. About one-third of all cases of hypertension are thought to be caused by obesity.

5. The risk of diabetes increases from twofold in those who are mildly overweight to tenfold in those who are severely obese.

6. Of individuals who lose weight, up to 95 percent will regain the weight in five years or less.

7. You can eat yourself to death.

It has been estimated that one-fourth to one-third of Americans are overweight, some 45 million people. Individuals who weigh 20 percent more than ideal body weight are considered obese.

Fig. 14.1 - Obesity Shape

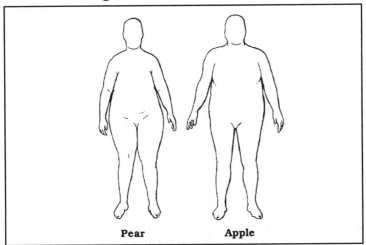

Pear   Apple

Distribution of excess weight, indicated by body shape (see Figure 14.1), is also important. Apple-shaped (top-heavy) bodies indicate that extra weight is centered around the waist; pear-shaped (bottom-heavy) bodies indicate that extra weight is centered on the hips and thighs. Of the two, apple-shaped bodies are more troublesome because they are associated with greater risks for:

- Heart disease
- Stroke
- High blood pressure
- Diabetes

Obesity can be found at all ages but is increasingly seen as individuals grow older and peaks at middle-age (see Figure 14.2). Studies suggest that up to 50 percent of those with a tendency to weight excess have some form of inherited predisposition. Other explanations for weight excess include:

- ○ The concept that a body mechanism, possibly controlled by genes, seeks a certain weight as if it were a set point for a given individual
- ○ Deficient exercise
- ○ Hormonal factors
- ○ Eating disorders (stress, depression, etc.)
- ○ Dietary factors, such as excess fat intake

In any case, weight gain occurs when calories taken in are greater than calories expended. Every 3,500 calories consumed in excess of those burned increase weight by about one pound. The reverse is true for weight loss.

It has been estimated that the average American consumes 3,700 calories per day, though only one-half that amount for women and two-thirds that amount for men is probably all that is needed for good body maintenance.

Being overweight and especially being obese have serious adverse consequences for health and longevity. Even a mild to moderate degree of weight excess can increase the risk of health complications and death at every age group.

Overweight people often have significant problems with blood fats (e.g., cholesterol and triglyceride levels), which partially explains the increased risk of coronary artery disease and the likelihood of heart attacks. Individuals who weigh 40 percent or more than ideal body weight are at increased risk for cancers of the:

- ○ Colon
- ○ Prostate

- Breast
- Gallbladder
- Kidney
- Stomach
- Uterus
- Ovary

One large study showed that women who gained more than 40 pounds after age 18 were three times more likely to have heart attacks than women who gained less than 12 pounds. Obesity is thought to be responsible for about one-third of all cases of high blood pressure.

High blood pressure in overweight people is also associated with an increased incidence of stroke and risks of developing:

- Diabetes
- Gallbladder disease
- Gout

Obesity can be associated with stresses on certain weight-bearing joints, resulting in arthritis and varying degrees of disability. Obesity, without other risk factors, may increase the likelihood of heart attack, especially for apple-shaped individuals.

In addition to known risk factors for cardiovascular disease, being of the male gender is associated with cardiovascular disease. In this regard, obesity in males is more of the apple-shape variety.

Overweight people also have more complications after surgery; wounds heal more slowly and infections are more common. Additionally, obesity is associated with:

- Anxiety
- Stress

- Depression
- Other consequences that affect quality and length of life

For improvement in quality and length of life, overweight/obese individuals should strive to achieve weights that are close to ideal for their age, sex, height, and build. A recent large study of nurses has put to rest concerns about adverse effects of thinness. That study showed that increased death rates thought to be present in very thin people were partly due to cigarette smoking or weight loss associated with cancers or other serious conditions.

It may be impossible for some individuals to reach desired weights, but even modest weight reduction has been associated with increased longevity and improved diabetes and high blood pressure control. Weight reduction can be achieved with the help of physicians or by team approaches (physicians, dietitians, and counselors).

Fig. 14.2 - Height/Weight Chart

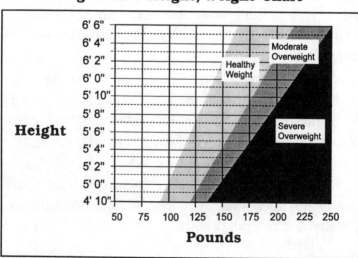

Dieting alone can help weight loss, but exercise provides additional benefits. Regular physical activity is especially important for weight maintenance. Physicians or psychiatrists/psychologists can assist with behavior modification programs.

Also, certain drugs can help in special situations. Physician-prescribed appetite suppressants, always combined with prudent diets, can provide superior weight loss results compared with diet therapy alone. However, some of diet medications have significant side effects, including an extremely rare form of irreversible high blood pressure in the pulmonary vessels. These medications should be used only under the direction of physicians. Pregnant women and individuals ages 65 and older should not initiate diets without consulting their physicians.

Recommendations

1. Try to achieve a weight close to ideal for your age, sex, build, height, and musculature.

2. Dieting, as suggested by your physician, and exercise should be the basis of any weight-loss program. This will work even if you have inherited a tendency toward obesity.

3. If you are unable to achieve ideal weight, lose as much weight as you can.

4. Avoid fad diets and medications or programs not approved by your physician.

5. Before initiating any weight loss program, determine if you have a medical condition (e.g., hypothyroidism, adrenal hormone excess, Cushing's syndrome, or kidney, heart, or liver

disease) that causes weight gain or if you take medications that contribute to weight gain (e.g., cortisone preparations).

Further Reading

Manson JE, Willett WC, Stampfer MJ, et al.: Body weight and mortality among women. New Eng J Med September 14, 1995.

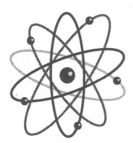

Alcohol:
Do Benefits Outweigh Dangers?

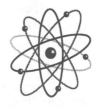

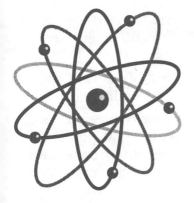

Eat not to dullness. Drink not to elevation.

-Benjamin Franklin

Facts

1. Alcohol-related deaths account for 2.7 million years of potential life lost annually in the U.S.; 65 percent of that loss is due to alcohol-related injuries.

2. People dying from alcohol-related causes lose an average of 26 years of normal life expectancy.

3. About one-third of drivers killed in vehicle crashes are intoxicated by alcohol.

4. The risk of dying in a traffic accident is eight times greater for heavy drinkers than for non-drinkers.

5. The risk of a fatal single-vehicle crash in drivers with a blood alcohol concentration of 0.09 percent (less than the common standard for driving legally, 0.10 percent) is 11.1 times greater than for nondrinkers. At blood alcohol concentrations of 0.15 percent or greater, the risk is 380 times greater.

6. Of those who kill themselves, 50 percent are intoxicated with alcohol or other drugs.

7. It appears that, in women, two to three drinks per day is associated with a 30-percent increase in breast cancer incidence or mortality; higher levels of alcohol consumption are associated with a 70-percent increase.

Alcohol is believed to be the most frequently abused drug throughout the world. It is associated with shortening life, as a prominent contributor to:

o   Death and debility from automobile accidents
o   Suicides
o   Other violent deaths

In the U.S. about 100,000 deaths each year are attributed to alcohol.

Additionally, liver cirrhosis, often a complication of alcoholism, is a relatively common cause of death among individuals ages 25 to 46. The presence of cirrhosis caused by alcohol considerably shortens expected lifespan. Significant alcohol ingestion over many years can result in severe heart problems and heart failure, and short-term heavy ingestion, such as in binge drinking, can lead to heart rhythm disturbances and even death.

Alcohol abuse also has been linked with cancers of the gastrointestinal and respiratory tracts and even the breast. Women who drink similar amounts as men appear to be more at risk for complications because they:

o   Appear to metabolize alcohol differently from men
o   Have a lower volume of body water
o   Reach a higher blood alcohol concentration in a shorter period of time with the same intake

Moderate drinking is defined as two drinks per day for men and one per day for women (a drink equals 12 oz. of regular beer, 5 oz. wine, or 1½ oz. of distilled spirits at 80-percent proof). One study found that ingestion of more than two drinks per day and progressively greater levels of consumption were associated with higher all-cause mortality.

Alcohol is also a problem for the elderly. Up to 10 percent of older adults living at home may have problems with alcohol. An even greater problem is seen in nursing homes. The elderly, because their body fluids are decreased, have higher blood alcohol levels and more complications than younger drinkers ingesting similar amounts of alcohol. Alcohol excess in the elderly can lead to various other problems, such as:

- Blood pressure elevation
- Depression
- Frequent falls
- Nutritional, vitamin, and mineral deficiencies
- Degenerative brain disorders
- Dementia

Because older adults often live alone, their drinking problems may not be recognized until major problems develop and mortality is high. Professional help is important in this group, whose responses to treatment are as good as those of younger drinkers.

Those who drink alcoholic beverages must determine their limitations of alcohol intake and maintain control of intake. Help in determining personal alcohol dependence can be obtained from answers to the CAGE questionnaire:

C - Have you considered **C**utting down on your drinking?

A - Have you ever become **A**ngry or **A**nnoyed about questions concerning your drinking?

G - Have you ever felt **G**uilty about your drinking practices?

E - Do you ever begin your day with an **E**ye opener?

Two or more yes answers suggest the likelihood of alcohol dependence; answering yes to all four strongly points to it. The recognition of alcohol dependence should be followed by treatment programs organized by personal physicians or special teams with recognized expertise.

People with family histories of alcoholism are at risk of becoming alcoholics themselves. In fact, drinkers with alcoholic parents are four times more likely to have problems with alcohol consumption than drinkers who have no family histories of alcohol problems.

The earlier alcohol dependence is detected and treated, the more likely it can be successfully treated and complications such as liver, heart, and neurological disorders can be avoided. As many as 50 percent of alcohol-dependent individuals do not recognize their disorder.

Another facet of alcohol ingestion must also be considered in view of recent findings. It appears that moderate consumption of alcohol (no more than two standard drinks daily for men and one for women) may be a reasonably good thing. Studies suggest that this consumption exerts a protective effect against coronary artery disease, which may lower heart disease risk by as much as 28 percent.

The mechanism for this beneficial effect could be its ability to elevate HDL cholesterol. A lot has been written about the type of alcohol that is most beneficial. In several regions of France, people eat diets rich in saturated fats and cholesterol but have low incidence of coronary artery disease, a situation termed the French Paradox.

Some researchers suggest that it is red wine, popular in France, that provides protection because red wine, unlike white, incorporates the skins of red grapes (which contain large amounts of phenolic compounds that behave like antioxidants) into the production process. Antioxidants, along with other substances in red wine that prevent blood clotting, may explain the reduction of coronary risk.

Other researchers feel that the ethanol itself causes the beneficial effect and that ethanol in red or white wine, beer, or other spirits could likely have the same effect. Many believe that other factors common to the French should also be considered, such as the increased amounts of fruits and vegetables (containing antioxidant vitamins) they consume or the fact that the French drink alcohol in moderation and with meals. Also, these groups dine differently than Americans, eating more heavily at midday than in the evening.

Other elements of the French or Mediterranean diet, such as olive oil and garlic, may also be important. It must be remembered, however, that the French, who boast the largest consumption of wine in the world, have much higher rates than other groups with lesser alcohol intakes of:

- Cirrhosis
- Upper gastrointestinal malignancies
- Accidents
- Suicides
- Violent deaths

Recommendations

1. If you don't drink, don't start.

2. If you wish to drink, some cardiac benefits may be derived from light to moderate drinking:
   - No more than two drinks daily for men
   - No more than one drink daily for women
   - No more than one drink daily for those ages 65 and older

3. Discuss openly your alcohol intake with your physician.

4. Individuals with concerns about breast or gastrointestinal cancers or strong family histories of alcoholism should discuss these situations with their physicians.

5. Some people should consider avoiding alcohol altogether, including:
   - Women who are pregnant or are trying to conceive
   - People who plan to drive or perform other activities that require unimpaired attention or muscular coordination
   - Individuals taking antihistamines, sedatives, or other medications that can magnify alcohol's effects
   - Recovering alcoholics
   - Persons being treated for anxiety or depression, since alcohol is thought to affect their clinical course and response to treatment adversely

Further Reading

Ewing JA: Detecting alcoholism: The CAGE questionnaire. JAMA 1984;252:1905-1907.

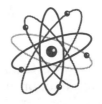

Stress and Depression:
Avoidance and Treatment as
Paths to Happiness

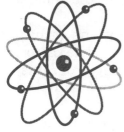

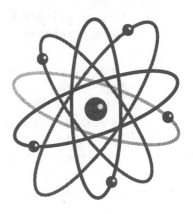

A vigorous five-mile walk will do more good for an unhappy but otherwise healthy adult than all the medicine and psychology in the world.

-Paul Dudley White

Facts

1. Primary care physicians treat depression and anxiety more than they treat heart disease, hypertension, or diabetes.
2. Up to 50 percent of patients with unexplained chest pains are really suffering from anxiety.
3. One-third of coronary artery patients have disease-related depression or anxiety.
4. About 25 percent of all suicides are committed by individuals ages 60 and older.
5. Depressed persons have suicide rates at least eight times higher than those of the general population.
6. Psychosocial stress interventions (group psychotherapy, counseling, relaxation training, and stress-reduction programs) reduce recurrent cardiac events (death and heart attacks) by 35 to 75 percent.
7. Pet owners have fewer risk factors for heart disease than individuals without such companions.
8. Depressed people have increased mortality from coronary artery disease and cancer.

9. Depression is common in smokers and alcohol dependents.
10. Up to two-thirds of persons with depression go undetected and untreated.
11. Depressive disorders occur in an estimated six percent of the general population but may be found in as many as 50 percent of those with medical illnesses.

At many points in life, individuals face various stresses of varying degrees. Such stresses can aggravate existing medical problems and possibly trigger new conditions. Various stressors have at times been associated with increased risks for heart attacks or strokes; these include:

- Anger
- Death of someone close
- Involvement in a war
- Being present during an earthquake or like catastrophe

Other stresses, especially when problems are ongoing, may lead to various problems from high blood pressure to cancer to sudden death; such stresses include:

- Major financial problems
- Significant family problems
- Loss of loved ones
- Unresolved grief
- Occupational stress
- Divorce
- Having certain diseases or physical problems

These responses to stresses and/or their complications can be associated with shortened lifespan. Stressful life events themselves can significantly increase the risk of death; these include:

- Divorce or separation
- Financial difficulty
- Being sued
- Insecure feelings at work

One interesting study showed that the risk

of heart attack increases 14-fold in the first 24 hours after the death of a loved one. By the end of the second day, the risk was still eight times higher than normal.

People who have family histories of depression or live particularly stressful lives are also prone to depression, especially if they:
- Have sudden, major life changes
- Are unmarried or widowed
- Lack supportive social networks
- Have certain physical conditions such as:
  - Cancer
  - Stroke
  - Heart disease
  - Dementia
  - Any chronic illness

One study has shown that death occurs several times more frequently in heart attack patients who also meet criteria for major depression in the six months after the event than those without depression.

Depression is also associated with biochemical disruptions in the brain, which fortunately respond to drug treatment. Drug treatment can also be effective in treating depression that results from stressful events.

Depression is common in American society, with about 15 percent of the population suffering from a major depressive disorder at some time in their lives. Unfortunately, this disorder is diagnosed and treated in fewer than one-third of these individuals. Among the elderly, major or minor depression is seen in about five percent of patients in primary care clinics and up to 25 percent of patients in nursing homes. Sadly, most elderly with depression fail to seek help. Moreover, depression can mimic dementia in the elderly.

Depressed individuals often have repeated visits to their physicians with complaints of:
- Vague pain
- Low energy
- Fatigue
- Insomnia
- Digestive problems
- Sexual difficulties

Physicians often fail to recognize symptoms of depression, which include:
- Persistent feelings of:
  - Sadness
  - Hopelessness
  - Pessimism
  - Anxiety
- Loss of interest or pleasure in ordinary activities, including sex
- Irritability
- Restlessness
- Decreased energy
- Fatigue
- Feeling slowed down
- Loss of appetite
- Weight loss
- Unintentional weight gain
- Sleeping too little or too much
- Difficulty with:
  - Concentration
  - Remembering
  - Making decisions
- Feelings of:
  - Guilt

- Worthlessness
- Helplessness
- Thoughts of death or suicide
- Suicide attempts
- Not caring whether one lives or dies from medical illness
- Excessive crying
- Recurrent aches and pains that do not respond to treatment
- Personality change
- Substance abuse

Of concern for all patients with depression is the possibility of suicide. Depression appears to be associated with about one-half of all suicides and is one of the strongest factors for attempted and completed suicides.

Suicide is a special problem in depressed older adults. About 25 percent of all suicides are committed by individuals ages 60 and older.

Depression is often a recurrent illness but can be treated effectively if it is recognized. Certain illicit drugs, alcohol, and prescription and non-prescription medicines can cause or complicate depression. Depression may also be a side effect of various medications or may be associated with numerous medical illnesses. Depression can also be related to seasonal decreases in the length of daylight, noted at both the northern and southern latitudes.

It has become clear that isolation from others is detrimental. Though data on the value of human connections are difficult to obtain, it appears that people with adequate social networks suffer less depression and live longer than those without such support systems. Valuable support system assets that allow and help people cope with stresses and complexities of life include:

- Friends
- Companions
- Acquaintances
- Comrades
- Spouses
- Associates
- Lovers
- Families
- Pets

Of untold value is belonging to such groups as:

- Religious communities
- Social networks
- Families
- Communities
- Sports teams

Recommendations

1. Do not be afraid to ask for help.

2. If you can eliminate, reduce, or modify stresses in your life, do so. Discussions of your stresses with physicians, psychiatrists/psychologists, or friends may help.

3. A routine exercise program often proves valuable for a variety of mental and emotional problems.

4. Maintain regular hours of adequate sleep (six to eight hours daily).

5. If you have symptoms of depression, seek your physician's help to sort out possible causes (drugs, illnesses, etc.) and start you on a treatment program.

6. Although thoughts of suicide are common in depression, such thoughts should encourage prompt consultation with your physician.

7. Develop and foster support groups in your life.

8. Do not drink alcohol if you are depressed or anxious or caffeine beverages if you are anxious; such drinks may increase anxiety.

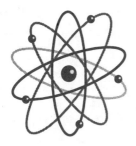

Immunizations: Increased Means of Disease Prevention

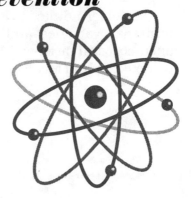

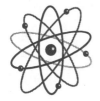

The value of life lies not in the length of days, but in the use we make of them. A man may live long yet live very little.

-Montaigne

Facts

1. Recent studies suggest epidemic-related pneumonia and influenza death rates among older adults, at between 50,000 and 70,000 annually.

2. Among older adults, only 52 percent receive influenza vaccines and 28 percent receive pneumococcal vaccines. These vaccines are free to Medicare and Medicaid beneficiaries.

Immunizations can reduce the incidence of major causes of disease, disability, and death in adults, especially in older populations. Routine vaccination programs can save lives with minimal effort expended.

INFLUENZA VACCINE

Most deaths from influenza virus infections occur in the elderly. In the U.S., 10,000 to 50,000 deaths each year have been associated with various epidemics. Vaccination from influenza results in:

- Less severe illness
- Lower fever
- Lower medical expenses
- Considerably lowered mortality

The U.S. Public Health Service recommends that influenza vaccines be given to all persons ages 65 and older as well as to younger persons in certain high-risk groups, including:

- Residents of chronic care facilities
- Individuals who suffer from chronic heart or lung disorders
- Individuals with chronic metabolic disease, such as:
  - Diabetes mellitus
  - Kidney dysfunction
  - Blood diseases
  - Lowered body immune resistance
- Individuals who travel to developing countries where medical care is less than optimal

The influenza vaccine prevents up to 80 percent of flu cases and an even higher percentage of flu-related deaths.

Vaccination of the staff in geriatric centers

is important and can reduce the mortality and influenza among patients in such facilities.

PNEUMOCOCCAL VACCINE

Pneumonia is the fifth leading cause of death in the elderly, with about one-third of adult pneumonia being caused by the pneumococcus bacteria. Mortality due to this infection is up to 10 times higher in elderly patients.

In recent years, strains of this bacteria have become resistant to usually effective antibiotics. The incidence of pneumococcal pneumonia is higher in:

- Nursing home residents
- Alcoholics
- Individuals with certain chronic medical conditions

Though statistics are difficult to interpret, studies suggest a protective value of pneumococcal vaccine in individuals with normal immune systems.

Possible benefits may be present for others, but most experts feel that rapidly emerging antibiotic resistance will soon mandate more aggressive vaccine programs to prevent pneumococcal pneumonia.

TETANUS VACCINE

In the U.S., tetanus, though rare, has become a disease of the elderly, with more than 50 percent of cases occurring in adults ages 60 and older and most of deaths occurring in patients ages 40 and older. Tetanus is found in individuals who have never received a completed vaccination series as a child. About 30 to 60 percent of adults ages 60 and older lack protective levels of tetanus antibodies. Death occurs in up to 24 percent of tetanus cases, with mortality being highest in the elderly.

Tetanus vaccination is effective. Although diphtheria is rare in the U.S., it is increasing in other countries; thus, the diphtheria vaccine is given along with tetanus.

HEPATITIS B VACCINE

Up to 300,000 individuals become infected with hepatitis B virus in the U.S. each year. Some of these individuals develop chronic active hepatitis and even cirrhosis. Complications of hepatitis B infection result in about 5,000 deaths per year in the U.S.

Hepatitis B is transmitted from person to person. The group at highest risk is intravenous drug users and their sex partners. Other high-risk groups include:

- Men who have sex with men
- Those with histories of sexual activity with multiple partners
- Travelers to high-risk areas
- Persons in health-related jobs who are exposed to blood or blood products
- Dialysis patients

Hepatitis B vaccine has proven to be effective.

HEPATITIS A VACCINE

Epidemics of hepatitis A are usually caused by fecally contaminated water or food; this is responsible for about one-half of cases in the U.S, at least 27,000 cases each year.

A certain small mortality is associated with

hepatitis A, but mortality increases with increasing age. Certain individuals are at higher risk for hepatitis A, including:

- Institutionalized persons and workers at such institutions
- Travelers to countries where hepatitis A is common
- Men who have sex with men
- Users of injection or street drugs
- Those in close contact with hepatitis A persons

The effectiveness of the newly available hepatitis A vaccine appears to be quite good.

Recommendations

1. Obtain the necessary immunizations at appropriate ages and keep immunizations current.

2. Travelers to Third World countries should consider having hepatitis vaccines.

Further Reading

Guide to Clinical Preventive Services, Report of the U.S. Preventive Services Task Force, 2nd ed. Williams & Wilkins 1996.

Diet:
What Are the Benefits of Fresh Fruits and Vegetables?

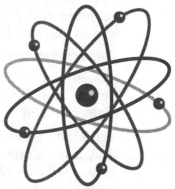

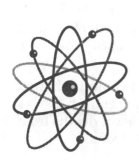

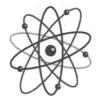

One should eat to live, not live to eat.

-Moliére

Facts

1. Studies suggest that reducing dietary fat to less than 30 percent of total calories can lower coronary artery disease mortality rates by as much as 20 percent.

2. Only about 20 percent of the U.S. population achieves the desired goal of 30 percent or less of calories from fat.

3. The average American's diet is 36 percent fat.

4. It is estimated that up to 50 percent of nursing home residents in the U.S. may be malnourished.

5. A recent large study of British subjects showed that daily consumption of fresh fruit was associated with significantly fewer deaths from coronary artery disease and stroke.

What you eat, how much you eat, and what you don't eat has important consequences to quality and length of life. It is important to establish healthy dietary patterns as early in life as possible and to maintain those patterns throughout life.

What is eaten influences the development of such problems as:

- High blood pressure
- Coronary artery disease
- Stroke
- Several different cancers
- Type II diabetes
- Gallbladder disease

Recent studies have shown that lowering cholesterol in the blood through drug therapy in people with histories of coronary artery disease or prior heart attack and elevated cholesterol definitely lengthened life. In this group, the risk of death from heart disease was 42 percent lower than for those untreated. Earlier studies by researchers such as Dean Ornish showed that coronary artery disease progression could be arrested and even reversed through programs of:

- Diet
- Exercise
- Stress reduction

Dr. Ornish currently is conducting a large multicenter study to confirm these observations. The diet in his program is rigorous but effective. It restricts fat intake to less than 10 percent of total calories, excluding all oils and animal products except for nonfat yogurt, skim milk, and egg whites. The program allows only 5 to 10 mg of dietary cholesterol daily.

This regimen contrasts with the American Heart Association program, which recommends no more than 30 percent of total calories from fat and daily cholesterol intake of less than 300 mg (one egg has about 215 mg of cholesterol).

Many experts feel that 30 percent of total calories as dietary fat is too high and that 20 to 25 percent is a more prudent figure. At present, the typical American diet is greater than 36 percent fat and at that level is sure to cause problems for certain individuals.

A prudent diet for most individuals is the dietary program endorsed by the American Heart Association (see Recommendations, below). Lack of response to that diet or lack of motivation to achieve better results with diet might make Dr. Ornish's program appealing.

In any case, working with physicians and skilled dietitians provides the best opportunity to find diets that are healthful and easy to follow.

At present, only about 20 percent of the U.S. population achieves the average daily goal of no more than 30 percent of calories from fat. Great importance should be attached to the amounts and types of fat in the diet.

Dietary fats are classified as saturated or unsaturated. Saturated fats are the most powerful dietary contributors to high blood cholesterol, particularly raising LDL in the blood. These fats present a special problem because they interfere with removal of cholesterol from the blood, which in turn results in elevation of blood cholesterol. Our bodies get along nicely without saturated fats in the diet because of the body's ability to produce them.

Unsaturated fats, found primarily in plants are of two kinds, monounsaturated and poly-unsaturated. When substituted for saturated fats in the diet, these fats can actually be associated with reducing LDL.

Examples of dietary fats are:

SATURATED	MONOUNSATURATED	POLYUNSATURATED
Butter	Avocado	Corn oil
Cheese	Canola oil	Cottonseed oil
Chocolate	Cashews	Margarine
Cocoa butter	Olives	Mayonnaise
Coconut	Olive oil	Pecans
Cream	Peanuts	Safflower oil
Egg yoke	Peanut butter	Soybean oil
Hydrogenated	Macadamia nuts	Sunflower seeds
oil	Hazelnuts	Walnuts
Lard	Pistachios	Pine nuts
Meat	Almonds	
Poultry		

Too much unsaturated fat in the diet can also increase the risk for heart disease and cancer.

Some individuals find it difficult to follow diet programs and resist formal programs proposed for them. In such cases, it may be better for physicians to provide these patients with basic guidelines for their eating. These may include:

 ○ Maintaining a desirable or ideal weight for your height
 ○ Eating less fat, especially animal fat and cholesterol
 ○ Eating less meat
 ○ Eating more plant foods, at least five portions of fruits and vegetables each day

Several studies have shown that individuals who eat large amounts of fruits and vegetables have lower risks of developing:

- High blood pressure
- Several cancers
- Strokes

A significant decrease in the risk of heart attack occurs as the amount of fiber in the diet is increased. Fiber can be found in:

- Fruits and vegetables
- Whole grains
- Beans
- Nuts
- Seeds
- Breads
- Pastas

High-fiber foods are also valuable because they tend to be filling; those offering the most fiber include:

- Grain foods, such as wheat bran cereal
- Fruits, such as stewed prunes
- Vegetables, such as broccoli

The U.S. Department of Agriculture recommends a diet program based on numbers of servings each day (based on caloric intake) from each of five food groups (see Figure 18.1).

Figure 18.1 - Food Guide Pyramid

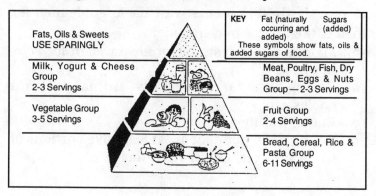

In the guide, the lower number of recommended servings is for the equivalent of a 1,600-calorie diet and the upper number for a 2,800-calorie diet.

The pyramid is an outline of what to eat each day rather than a rigid prescription. It calls for eating a variety of foods to get needed nutrients. Foods in one group cannot replace those in another.

The value of fruits and vegetables in the diet is becoming more apparent; not only are they helpful in avoiding coronary artery disease but they also have a place in cancer prevention. The National Cancer Institute supports a program that includes eating five or more servings of fruits and vegetables per day as part of a low-fat, high-fiber diet. Studies show that less than one-third of the population actually achieves this goal and that the majority of people consume less than one serving of fruit per day. Worse yet, only about one-fourth of the population is aware of this dietary recommendation.

Some people are confused by the recommendations for fruits and vegetables. A recent British Medical Journal article helps clarify some of these concerns. The authors recommend eating a wide variety of fruits and vegetables, allowing in this category the inclusion of such items as:

- Fruit juice
- Baked beans
- Dried fruit
- Frozen and canned fruit
- Vegetables and fruits as found in pies

They exclude:

- Potatoes
- Fruit drinks
- Nuts

They also clarify the meaning of a serving or portion in a way that is more readily understood:

FOOD TYPE	PORTION (Serving)*	EXAMPLE
FRUIT		
Very large fruit	One large slice	Melon, pineapple
Large fruit	One whole	Apple, banana
Medium fruit	Two whole	Plum, kiwi
Berries	Cupful	Raspberries, grapes
Stewed/canned fruit	Three serving spoonfuls	Stewed apple,
Dried fruit	Half serving spoonful	canned peaches
Fruit juice	Full wine glass	Apricots, raisins
		Orange juice, fresh
VEGETABLES		
Green vegetables	Two serving spoonfuls	Broccoli, spinach
Root vegetables	Two serving spoonfuls	Carrots, parsnip
Very small vegetables	Three serving spoonfuls	Peas, sweet corn
Pulses and beans	Two serving spoonfuls	Baked beans,
Salad	Bowlful	kidney beans
		Lettuce, tomato

*A portion is equal to approximately 80 grams or almost 3 ounces. From British Medical Journal 1995;310.

Currently there is a definite movement away from meat and toward vegetarian diets. Studies show that those eating meatless diets have much lower risks of dying from cancer or from any cause. Nutritionally sound vegetarian diets have definite benefits over diets that include animal foods. Several variations of strict vegetarian diets are both attractive and healthful.

WHAT ABOUT OTHER ITEMS IN THE DIET?
SODIUM

The body actually needs very little sodium (less than one-fourth teaspoon) each day. It appears reasonable to avoid excess salt in the diet, especially if blood pressure levels are borderline or elevated. Salt is also a problem for the obese and those who tend to retain fluids.

SOY PROTEIN

Tofu, soy flour, etc. may have value when eaten in combination with prudent diets. More information about soy proteins is needed.

OLIVE OIL

Olive oil is a valued and tasty replacement for butter and meat but has 120 calories per tablespoon.

GARLIC, OAT BRAN, PSYLLIUM, NUTS

Garlic, oat bran, psyllium, and nuts are probably all effective to some degree in conjunction with a low-fat diet.

COFFEE

Coffee probably is not much of a risk if no more than five cups per day are consumed unless individuals have special sensitivities to caffeine products.

Recommendations

1. Follow a dietary program that allows you to maintain desirable weight.

2. Familiarize yourself with the Food Guide Pyramid.

3. Reduce meat and fat in your diet.

4. Eat at least five portions of fruits and vegetables each day.

5. Whenever possible, substitute unsaturated for saturated fat.

Recommendations from the American Heart Association

The American Heart Association recommends that those with elevated blood cholesterol levels follow a Step I or Step II diet as advised by their physicians.

STEP I DIET

On a Step I diet, patients should eat:

- 30 percent or less daily total calories from fat
- Eight to 10 percent daily total calories from saturated fat
- Less than 300 mg of dietary cholesterol per day
- Just enough calories to achieve and maintain healthy weight. (The physician or dietitian can determine an individual's reasonable calorie level)

Patients whose blood cholesterol levels are not lowered sufficiently using the Step I diet or who are at high risk for heart disease should switch to the Step II diet. Patients with heart disease should start with the Step II diet.

STEP II DIET

On a Step II diet, patients should eat:

- Less than seven percent daily total calories from saturated fat
- 30 percent or less daily total calories from fat
- Less than 200 mg of dietary cholesterol per day
- Just enough calories to achieve and maintain a health weight. (The physician or dietitian can determine an individual's reasonable calorie level)

Further Reading

Williams C: Healthy eating: Clarifying advice about fruits and vegetables. Br Med J 1995;310.

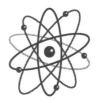

Exercise:
Physical and Mental Benefits

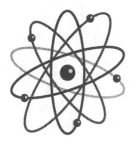

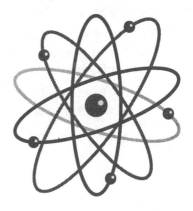

If we could give every individual the right amount of exercise, not too little and not too much, we would have found the safest way to health.

-Hippocrates

Facts

1. About 24 percent of Americans ages 18 and older report no leisure-time physical activity.

2. Among people ages 55 and older, 38 percent report essentially sedentary lifestyles.

3. It has been estimated that about 12 percent of all mortality in the U.S. is related to lack of regular physical activity.

4. Regular strenuous leisure time exercise in middle-aged men can decrease the risk of cardiac arrest by up to 65 percent and that of sudden heart attack by up to 30 percent.

5. Exercise can reduce total mortality and cardiac mortality by 20 to 25 percent in patients with coronary artery disease.

6. A routine exercise program has proven valuable for a variety of mental and emotional problems.

7. Estimates suggest that only about 38 percent of women exercise regularly.

Each year in the U.S., as many as 250,000 deaths are attributed to lack of regular physical activity. Many studies have shown that physical activity reduces the risk of many diseases such as:

- Heart disease
- High blood pressure
- Cancer
- Osteoporosis
- Diabetes mellitus

The exact manner in which exercise exerts its many beneficial effects is unknown, but important associations and long-term benefits of exercise have been recognized and confirmed. Exercise has been associated with lower blood pressure and improved blood fat profiles than are found for sedentary individuals. Exercise:

- Increases HDL cholesterol levels
- Lowers triglyceride levels
- Sometimes decreases LDL cholesterol levels

It also appears to be able to delay onset of heart disease and, should heart attack occur, improve survival rates. The risk of heart attack was reduced by as much as 50 percent in active compared to sedentary men.

In a London study of middle-aged conductors of double-decker busses, conductors who constantly ran from the lower to upper decks and down again had smaller waist sizes and developed much less coronary artery disease than sedentary bus drivers.

Exercise also appears to be able to reduce risks of potentially dangerous blood clots forming in the body under certain conditions and of heart irregularities by other mechanisms. It can also improve functional work capacity and help control body weight.

For many years, physical inactivity had been recognized as a contributor to development of coronary artery disease. More recently, however, a sedentary lifestyle has been noted as a major risk factor for coronary artery disease, along with other risk factors, including:

o High blood pressure
o Hypercholesterolemia
o Cigarette smoking

Though most earlier studies were conducted with male subjects, recent studies suggest that physical activity also offers cardiovascular protection for women. One study found a 44-percent reduction in risk of heart attack associated with regular exercise in women. Recent studies have also suggested that elderly subjects who exercised developed disability at a much slower rate than those who did not, despite the fact that those who exercised had higher rates of fractures and short-term problems related to exercise behaviors. Those in the exercise group also had lower mortality.

The benefits of exercise are not limited to the heart. Patients with peripheral vascular disease can significantly improve their walking ability with exercise programs. Studies show that exercise protects against:

o Colon cancer
o Development of noninsulin-dependent diabetes
o Osteoporosis
o Mental health disorders

The problem of lack of exercise is particularly important in the U.S. where it includes 20 to 30 percent of the population. This indicates that 35 to 50 million Americans are at a two to four fold increased risk for cardiovascular mortality. Only about 22 percent of American adults meets or exceeds recently recommended exercise guidelines. About 54 percent is involved in some physical activity but not enough to meet the guidelines; 24 percent is sedentary and does little if any exercise. In the latter group, it has been estimated that as much as 35 percent of excess coronary artery disease could be eliminated if these people became more physically active.

The question is how much exercise is enough? Current recommendations from the Centers for Disease Control and Prevention and the American College of Sports Medicine are that every adult in the U.S. accumulate about 30 minutes of moderately intense physical activity preferably every day. This can be accomplished in one effort or from several shorter bouts of activity during the course of a day. A brisk walk (at a rate of three to four miles per hour) is a good standard. Other activities, such as dancing, climbing stairs, and cycling can be substituted according to personal desires and preferences. The goal is to expend at least 200 extra calories each day by exercise.

Many books and pamphlets commercially available can translate the amount or length of a favorite activity that is necessary to fulfill recommended exercise guidelines (e.g., 20 minutes of jogging burns about 200 calories). Current exercise recommendations are considered minimum suggestions. It appears that the more exercise performed, within reason, the better and the lower the risk of disability and death from coronary artery disease.

A recent report from Stanford University suggests that older persons ages 50 to 72 who engage in vigorous running and other aerobic activities have lower mortality and slower development of disability than members of the general population. Exercise and strength-training sessions have been shown to be beneficial even for the very elderly, ages 75 and older. It is the hope that such activities for these people will result in:

- Improved:
  - Ambulation
  - Balance
  - Coordination
- Fewer falls
- Better ability to maintain independent lifestyles

Some have expressed concerns about possible development of cardiac problems during vigorous exercise; however, about 96 percent of heart attacks occur during rest, with only four percent related to vigorous exertion. Also, of those who have heart attacks during vigorous exertion, the majority had been sedentary or were among those who exercised infrequently. Those who exercised regularly had an overall lower risk of heart attack.

Recommendations

1. Walk briskly for at least one-half hour six to seven days a week.
2. Continue an exercise program throughout your life.

3. If you have medical problems, disabilities, or other limitations, seek a physician's advice and guidance in initiating and developing an exercise program.

4. If you are able, choose a more vigorous physical activity program for added benefits.

5. Even if you are unable to increase activity to desired or recommended levels, any increase in activity is beneficial and can reduce the risk of coronary artery disease.

6. Seek activities you enjoy; you are more likely to stick with them.

Further Reading

Fries JF, Singh G, et al.: Running and the development of disability with age. Ann Int Med October 1994.

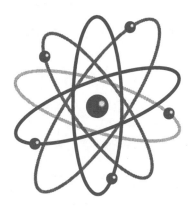

Sleep:
Importance to Personal Health

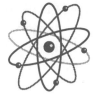

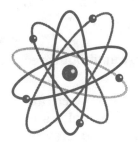

Sleeping is no mean art. For its sake one must stay awake all day.

-Neitzsche

Facts

1. Up to five percent of middle-aged men have sleep apnea.

2. Automobile accidents occur about two to three times more often in individuals with sleep apnea.

3. The incidence of heart attack is about five times greater in patients who snore and have sleep apnea.

4. Individuals with sleep apnea are at about three times greater risk of stroke.

5. Studies have shown that cigarette smokers are significantly more likely than nonsmokers to report problems going to sleep and staying asleep and daytime sleepiness.

Sleep occupies a significant portion of the average day. At some time or other, most people have complaints of difficulty falling asleep and staying asleep or not feeling rested after sleep. Some people feel excessively sleepy during the day without realizing that something might be wrong with their sleep.

Transient problems with sleep, often associated with various identifiable factors, are recognized and usually managed by individuals. Chronic problems, however, often are undiagnosed and thus untreated. Their importance is unrecognized and thus do not get reported to physicians.

It is a common thing for individuals to fall asleep while driving and become involved in traffic accidents. Probably most of these victims are healthy people who are sleep-deprived due to lifestyle or work schedules, though many of them may have long-standing sleep disorders (such as sleep apnea) that interfere with sleep on a regular basis and cause subsequent loss of daytime alertness and increased risks of automobile accidents. Also, some may be taking medications that have sedating effects or that disrupt routine sleeping patterns.

Patients must discuss sleep problems with their physicians. Sleep complaints suggest several important causes, including:

- Psychiatric illnesses (often depression)
- Major medical illnesses, especially those involving the:
  - Thyroid gland
  - Heart
  - Lung

A large variety of nonprescription and prescription drugs can interfere with sleep; these include:

- Nonprescription (over-the-counter):
  - Pseudoephedrine
  - Phenylpropanolamine
  - Diphenhydramine
  - Chlorpheniramine
- Prescription:
  - Antidepressants (amitriptyline, doxepin)
  - Propranolol
  - Metoprolol
  - Clonidine

This side effect may occur only in some individuals or under certain circumstances and thus may not have been anticipated. Alcohol, caffeine, and even some medications thought to help sleep can cause problems with sleep for certain individuals.

Sleep problems are even more common in the elderly and become more prominent with advancing age. Older individuals can be bothered during the day with:

- Fatigue
- Impaired thinking
- Decline in motor skill capabilities
- Decreased alertness

These effects are problematic when this or any population drives a car or works with potentially dangerous machinery. Reasonable estimates suggest that about 15 to 20 percent of all motor vehicle accidents are attributable to sleepiness. In the U.S., this would amount to up to 7,000 fatalities per year.

The most serious sleeping disorder is sleep apnea, a relatively common disorder seen in about two percent of women and four percent of men (about two to five million people in the U.S.). In sleep apnea individuals stop breathing up to hundreds of times each night during sleep. An excess of 10 such events per hour are generally necessary to establish diagnosis. These individuals are often unaware of their problem and often do not suspect any sleep problem.

Sleep apnea tends to be more common in the elderly (some degree of it occurs in 25 percent of people ages 60 and older) and in association with obesity and high blood pressure. Certain airway obstruction problems may be found in such individuals.

Symptoms of sleep apnea include:

- Snoring
- Daytime sleepiness
- Early morning headache
- Memory changes
- Thought deficits
- Depression

These symptoms often are overlooked, though loud snoring, choking noises, and disruptions of breathing noted by sleeping partners may be the best clue to sleep apnea.

As occurs with other sleep disorders, sleep apnea patients have a higher frequency of automobile accidents. More important problems, however, result from poor oxygenation of the blood during periods of disrupted breathing, including:

- Heart attack
- Stroke
- Sudden death

Complicating the ability to diagnose sleep apnea is the fact that symptoms often are misinterpreted as anxiety or depression or the results of aging. Additionally, many physicians are unfamiliar with the disorder and the varied and confusing forms that it can manifest.

There are specific, effective, and often lifesaving treatments for sleep apnea and the diseases that may be associated with it.

Recommendations

1. Recognize that sleep disorders exist and can have serious consequences.

2. Recognize that lifestyle factors (smoking, alcohol, drugs) can interfere with sleep.

3. Seek your partner's observations of your nighttime snoring or breathing habits.

4. Be suspicious of any medications you take as possible causes or contributors to sleeping disorders.

5. If you are suspicious of sleep apnea, avoid sleeping on your back; elevating the head of the bed may also help.

6. Any suspicion of a sleep disorder should be brought to the attention of a physician who is knowledgeable about and interested in the condition.

7. Lack of response to therapies, suspicion of repeated sleep disorder-related accidents, or a picture suggesting sleep apnea or its complications should trigger a request for an evaluation at a recognized sleep disorder center.

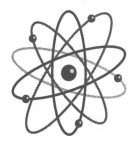

Vitamins and Supplements:
Which Are Necessary for Health?

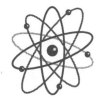

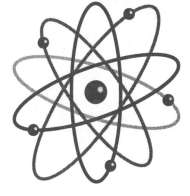

Life loves to be taken by the lapels and told, "I am with you, kid. Let's go."

-Maya Angelou

Facts

1. Many Americans take vitamin supplements, though most do not need them.
2. Vitamins taken in excess of the Recommended Daily Allowances can be harmful.
3. Mineral requirements can easily be met with a balanced, varied diet.

Millions of Americans take vitamin and mineral supplements, responding to suggestions by supplement manufacturers that their products can prolong life, increase energy, prevent cancers and heart disease, improve sexual prowess, and ward off disease. Guidelines for vitamin requirements are set by the Food and Nutrition Board of the National Research Council and termed Recommended Dietary Allowances (RDAs). These recommendations exceed the needs of most healthy people but avoid excesses that can be potentially harmful.

Barrett and Herbert in their book *The Vitamin Pushers* suggest only two situations in which vitamin use in excess of RDAs has proven of value. The first is for treatment of medically diagnosed deficiency states, rare except among alcoholics, persons with intestinal absorption problems, and the poor, especially those who are pregnant or elderly. The second situation is in the treatment of certain rare conditions for which large doses of vitamins are used as drugs, with full recognition of the risks involved.

Most adults should not require supplements because they probably obtain adequate nutrient intake from their diets. Essential nutrients can be obtained from balanced and varied diets that contain:
- Lots of fruits and vegetables
- Grains
- Some dairy products
- Lean meat
- Skinless poultry
- Fish

Obtaining necessary nutrients from the diet avoids problems related to excess vitamin and mineral intake yet provides the various known and unknown materials in foods that assist and/or supplement the actions of vitamins, minerals, and other materials found in foods.

Significant problems can result from excessive doses of:

- Vitamin A
- Vitamin C
- Vitamin E
- Folate
- Vitamin B_6
- Niacin
- Selenium
- Zinc
- Calcium
- Iron

Some people do need a multiple vitamin/mineral supplement on a daily basis. Supplements are safe if they contain no more than 150 percent of RDAs for each component. Individuals most likely to benefit from daily multiple vitamin/mineral supplements include:

- Dieters with fewer than 1,200 calories daily
- Individuals with malabsorption syndromes
- Elderly people who:
  - Appear malnourished
  - Have poor diets
  - Have poor appetites
- Individuals with specific vitamin or mineral deficiencies as suggested by a manifest disease process
- Alcoholics
- Smokers

- Pregnant and nursing women
- Individuals taking drugs that distort the appetite
- Strict vegetarians
- Individuals with kidney failure, especially if on dialysis
- Elderly people with poor sunlight exposure
- Most postmenopausal women, who need calcium supplements
- Menstruating women, who may need iron supplements

Much interest has been generated by the possibility that beta carotene and vitamins C and E may help prevent cancer and heart disease because of their antioxidant qualities. At present, however, the best recommendation is to include more of the natural foods (mostly fruits, vegetables, and grains) that contain antioxidants in the diet.

The value of dietary enhancements is noted in important studies done at Harvard and the University of Texas, which showed that individuals who ate the equivalent of one to one and one-half carrots a day for lengthy periods had more than a 20-percent lower risk of death from all causes and an equally lower risk of heart disease in women when compared with those who ate the least amount of beta carotene in their diets. At the same time, beta carotene supplements have not shown any mortality reduction benefits with regard to cancer, heart disease, or other causes.

Despite numerous and varied claims for mineral supplements, healthy people eating an appropriate number of calories in varied diets with plenty of fruits, vegetables, and grains can easily achieve the recommended intake of minerals. These minerals include:

- ○ Calcium
- ○ Selenium
- ○ Iron
- ○ Zinc
- ○ Chromium
- ○ Iodine
- ○ Phosphorus
- ○ Cobalt
- ○ Copper
- ○ Fluoride
- ○ Manganese
- ○ Molybdenum

Taken in excess, individual minerals or combinations of them can cause problems, including toxicity. Such is not expected from ingesting minerals in natural food sources.

The exception to this rule is calcium. To protect against osteoporosis, increased incidence of fractures in the elderly, and associated increased mortality, calcium supplements may be required. The elderly, due to dietary deficiencies and/or lack of sunlight exposure may be deficient in calcium and vitamin D. (See Section #6 for recommended dosages of calcium supplements.) Dairy products, such as skim milk (300 mg calcium per cup), are the best source of dietary calcium. For those unable to ingest enough dietary calcium, supplements, such as calcium carbonate or calcium citrate taken two or three times daily with meals, is beneficial. In the elderly with poor sun exposure, the addition of 200 to 400 IU of vitamin D should prove helpful.

It is amazing what individuals are willing to ingest in efforts to achieve healthier and longer lives, avoid problems associated with natural aging, and restore qualities and feelings associated with youth. Manufacturers of so-called supplements, health foods, and natural products claim benefits for which there are no supporting evidence, no FDA-approval, and usually no scientific basis. Often these items are expensive and by themselves can be dangerous or prove to be especially toxic when combined with other drugs or items ingested. Additionally, physicians are unaware of problems associated with long-term ingestion of these items; no lists include all items that fall into this category. Popular substances currently are:

- DHEA
- Chromium picolinate
- Coenzyme Q_{10}
- Comfrey
- Ginkgo biloba
- Ginseng
- Ma huang
- Melatonin (when used for other than sleep disorders)

The authors advise avoiding these and all other unapproved items, since none has ever reached the stature, scientific acceptance and approval, or cost effectiveness gained simply by eating five servings of fruits and vegetables.

Recommendations

1. Obtain vitamins and minerals from a balanced diet that includes at least five servings of fruits, vegetables, and grains daily.

2. A simple, inexpensive multiple vitamin/mineral supplement based on RDAs benefit certain groups (see above).

3. Avoid vitamin/mineral supplements in dosages above RDAs.

4. You may need calcium supplements, depending on your age, gender, and dietary calcium intake.

5. Barrett and Herbert (see below) soundly suggest that "the most prudent course of action is to forget about using herbs for medicinal purposes."

Further Reading

Barrett S, Herbert V: *The Vitamin Pushers.* Prometheus Books, 1994.

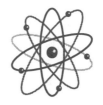

Aspirin: The Magic Potion?

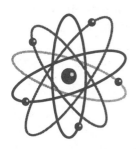

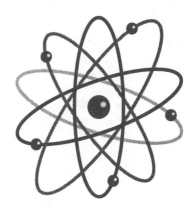

The desire to take medicine is perhaps the greatest feature which distinguishes man from animals.

-William Osler

Facts

1. For those who have had heart attacks, aspirin could reduce the risk of having another by 30 percent.

2. It appears that people who take aspirin are less likely to die from cancers of the colon, rectum, stomach, and esophagus.

Aspirin is an important drug with many uses. Potential beneficial effects of aspirin intake in people with heart disease, stroke, and certain blood vessel problems and people who might develop certain cancers suggest a role for this drug in life extension.

Though aspirin has many potential beneficial effects, its widespread usage is limited by a variety of significant side effects that include:

- Peptic ulcers
- Gastritis
- Hemorrhage in the:
  - Upper gastrointestinal tract
  - Urinary tract
  - Bowel
  - Brain
- Allergic reactions (occasionally)

A recent study suggests that there is no significant difference in the rates of upper gastrointestinal bleeding with the use of regular aspirin or the more expensive enteric-coated or buffered form.   Aspirin can also be a problem for those with uncontrolled hypertension and for alcoholics because of hemorrhagic strokes and gastrointestinal bleeding, respectively.

Aspirin is effective for those with coronary artery disease and those who have had or are at increased risk for heart attack. It is especially useful in lowering risk of death (by 15 percent) and heart attack in patients in the process of having heart attacks.

Use of aspirin in middle-aged or older men who, because of risk factors, are at great risk for a first heart attack may be beneficial, but potential side effects may negate the desired value. In men without symptoms or risk factors for coronary artery disease, aspirin may prove more harmful than beneficial. If used, probably low-dose (one baby aspirin) each day taken with food will provide benefit while minimizing risks.

Studies have shown a benefit of aspirin in reducing the risk of stroke in patients with symptoms (transient ischemic attacks [TIAs] or stroke) but not much benefit in asymptomatic individuals. Aspirin may have some benefit in reducing stroke associated with certain heart rhythm disorders (e.g., atrial fibrillation).

Aspirin appears to have some anticancer effects in the digestive tract, especially the large bowel, when taken for many years. The data are still not strong enough, however, in view of potential aspirin complications, to recommend routine use for this purpose.

Recommendations

1. Take aspirin (dose as recommended by your physician) if you have coronary artery disease and especially if you have poorly controlled symptoms of same or have had a heart attack.

2. Take aspirin if you have symptoms or signs suggesting an impending stroke (TIA) or after a completed stroke.

3. Avoid aspirin if you are already taking other blood thinners, have or are prone to peptic ulcers, or have other potential bleeding problems.

4. Use the lowest dose of aspirin that is known to be effective for the condition under treatment.

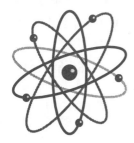

Estrogen and Progesterone: Benefits and Dangers

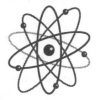

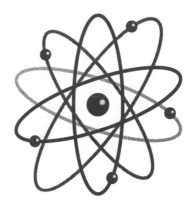

There is a fountain of youth: it is your mind, your talents, the creativity you bring to your life and the lives of people you love. When you learn to tap this resource, you will truly have defeated old age.

-Sophia Loren

Facts

1. Estrogen replacement therapy can reduce the risk of coronary artery disease by as much as 50 percent.

2. Estrogen replacement therapy could reduce the risk of hip fracture in women by as much as 25 to 50 percent.

3. Studies suggest that smoking has an anti-estrogen effect.

4. A recent study suggests that estrogen may delay onset and decrease risks of Alzheimer's disease in postmenopausal women.

With vast numbers of women at or approaching menopause, it is important to consider interventions that might reduce or prevent long-term effects of estrogen deficiency, namely coronary artery disease and osteoporosis. After menopause, blood fat patterns change significantly, with increases in LDL and decreases in HDL cholesterol levels. These and other changes can eventually result in the development of coronary artery disease that will occur in about one-half these women in their lifetimes, with about 30 percent dying from it. Estrogen should be considered a first-line agent for reducing LDL cholesterol and raising HDL cholesterol.

Declining estrogen levels in postmenopausal women result in hundreds of thousands of osteoporosis-related fractures. These hip and spine fractures, which can be crippling, occur in about one-half of all postmenopausal women who live into their 80s. Estrogen replacement therapy could reduce the risk of hip fracture in women by as much as 25 to 50 percent. Women most likely to benefit from estrogen are those:

- With early or surgical menopause
- With multiple cardiac risk factors, especially blood fat abnormalities
- At increased risk for osteoporosis or fractures, such as those who:
  - Smoke
  - Have family histories of fractures
  - Are thin
  - Have been on lengthy courses of cortisone preparations

Some women should not have estrogen therapy. This group includes women with prior breast cancer and histories of estrogen-related complications or liver disease.

There are some side effects of estrogen therapy. These include endometrial cancer if estrogen is given without progesterone and a possible increased risk of breast cancer. Counseling and close follow-up by physicians is necessary for the length of estrogen treatment programs, especially for women who have not had hysterectomies.

For women who have had hysterectomies, estrogen is best used alone. Uterine cancer occurs in about 2.6 percent of white women ages 50 and older. Estrogen use in postmenopausal women significantly increases risks of uterine cancer, that risk increasing with dose and duration of treatment.

Progesterone, often given with estrogen in women who still have uteri, eliminates excess risk of uterine cancer. The possible and controversial small increase in risk of breast cancer with estrogen alone is basically unchanged by adding progesterone, despite earlier thoughts that progesterone might be protective.

Progesterone is commonly associated with what are often considered to be transient side effects such as:
- Headache
- Bloating
- Irritability
- Depression
- Vaginal bleeding and related problems

There was also concern that the addition of progesterone might blunt the cardioprotective effects of estrogen therapy. Recent reports, however, suggest that adding progesterone to estrogen therapy does not appear to do so in relatively young postmenopausal women.

Recommendations

1. At the time of menopause, ask your physician about particular benefits and risks from estrogen replacement therapy for you.

2. If you are not a good candidate for estrogen replacement therapy, learn about and institute alternative regimens for avoiding osteoporosis and for reducing your risks for coronary artery disease.

3. You can begin estrogen replacement therapy even if you are in your 70s.

4. For the greatest benefit, continue estrogen replacement therapy for the long-term.

5. If you are postmenopausal with coronary artery disease, estrogen replacement may have added value for you.

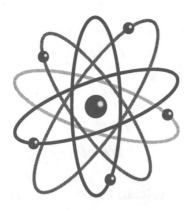

The Physician:
How to Select Your Doctor

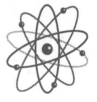

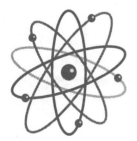

A physician can sometimes parry the scythe of death, but has no power over the sand in the hour-glass.

-Hester Lynch Piozzi

Fact

1. A quality physician could prove to be one of the most important variables influencing life extension.

There is little doubt that good physicians involved in good physician/patient relationships can influence the extension of life, and the quality of that extended life should also be improved.

Much care should go into selection of personal physicians. People want physicians with whom they can feel compatible in relationships that will last for many years. Personal physicians usually are internists or family physicians. Patients must take time to find physicians they like and trust and with whom they have a good personality match.

Sometimes recommendations from friends and relatives, or especially other physicians, can put patients in contact with doctors who can be considered for the important task of overseeing health. Patients should seek physicians who, from the beginning, seem interested in them, their problems, and health maintenance. Physicians should be willing to spend a reasonable amount of time with patients during visits; after visits, patients should feel that their problems have been heard.

Obviously, patients should expect to be tended by quality physicians with excellent reputations. Patients should feel free to check credentials of candidates.

Some may desire doctors who are listed in Best Doctors in America or similar publications; these physicians are often found at major university medical centers, but they often have restricted practices because of teaching and research commitments. In recent years, however, many of these doctors have become more involved in patients' clinical care.

In seeking the right physicians, patients might consider their own special needs and specialty side interests and skills of physician candidates. For example, internists with subspecialty interests in endocrinology might be the best match for diabetic patients. Primary physicians, however, can always direct patients to capable specialists needed to manage special problems.

Patients should note whether their personal physicians stay current with medical practices and research. This discovery will only occur with time, however, as patients determine whether they are receiving the benefits of the latest technological advances, treatments, and medicines and whether their physicians can answer questions about current media reports. It should be recognized, however, that the media often overwhelm the public with frequent reports of unimportant but interest-generating medical findings or studies. Good physicians, however, will seek pertinent information and put it into proper perspective regarding their patients' illnesses and needs.

There are numerous ways in which a physician's care can improve the quality and length of life. Good physicians will:

- Oversee patients' immunization programs, thus preventing sometimes serious or life-shortening illnesses

- Ensure proper screening studies and examinations to discover diseases at early stages when they are easier to treat

- Upon hearing patients' symptoms, quickly pursue problems and institute therapies early and effectively

- Avoid unnecessary and/or dangerous testing or procedures

- Use tried and tested medicines and treatments, always cognizant of side effects and complications

- Be concerned about potential problems related to combinations of drugs used in treating patients' problems

- Choose the best available consulting, surgical, or other procedure-performing specialists in an effort to achieve the best results for their patients

- Help their patients select the best hospitals, care centers, or emergency units if needed

- Guide their patients to the most effective therapy centers, rehabilitation units, and dietary and lifestyle modification programs

- Confront their patients regularly about issues such as smoking, alcohol, safe sex, exercise, and cardiovascular risk factors

- Be interested in cost factors associated with evaluation and treatment, recognizing that cost-effectiveness considerations must be part of their patients' care

- Be interested in their patients' total spectrum of problems, such as anxiety, depression, or dementia, since these can trigger, mimic, cause, or exacerbate numerous other problems and result in unwanted or unexpected outcomes (suicide, accidents, etc.)

- Be advocates working in their patients' behalf when conflicts arise with health management organizations (HMOs) or other managed-care entities

- Guarantee that their practice coverage for nights, weekends, vacations, etc. is by qualified individuals who are able to meet patients' healthcare needs

It is important that there be a cooperative, understanding physician/patient relationship in order that patients might derive the greatest benefit from the association. Patients sometimes desire frequencies of visits/examinations, tests or procedures, medications, or therapies that physicians may feel are inappropriate, cost-ineffective, or potentially harmful. Today especially, physicians try to keep people out of expensive hospital settings when reasonable alternatives are available, but physicians should be willing to discuss with their patients the particular care options.

As important as it is to find good physicians and establish effective physician/patient relationships, it is equally important that patients be cautious about alternative practices that claim effectiveness beyond proven demonstration of their utility. The use of alternative therapies to treat serious, life-threatening conditions can be catastrophic. Though large numbers and varieties of these therapies exist, a few are worthy of mention:

- Homeopathy - The use of remedies prepared by extreme dilutions of natural substances such as plants and minerals to treat diseases. These remedies are generally ineffective because the concentrations of substances are inadequate for biological activity

- Acupuncture - A form of Chinese medicine associated with the insertion of fine needles under the skin at specified points in the body for treatment of various problems and diseases. With the possible exception of pain management and substance abuse treatment, acupuncture should not be substituted for proven therapies for treatment of significant illnesses

○ Chelation therapy - A synthetic amino acid, EDTA, and other substances given intravenously to patients who seek relief from coronary artery disease, atherosclerosis, peripheral vascular disease, and a host of other major and minor illnesses. Of concern is that cardiac patients undergoing such treatments are in great need of effective, standard, proven therapy rather than this unproven approach

Recommendations

1. Use the information suggested in this chapter and take the time and effort to find the best physician match for your particular needs.

2. Beware of alternative practices and approaches to treatment that appear to offer simple solutions to major medical problems.

Further Reading

Barrett S and Herbert V: *The Vitamin Pushers.* Prometheus Books, Amherst, N.Y., 1994.

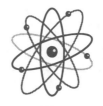

The Patient: Personal Responsibility for Wellness

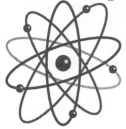

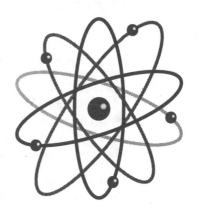

The patient must combat the disease with the physician.

-Hippocrates

Facts

1. One-third of women who are prescribed estrogen replacement therapy never fill their prescriptions.

2. Of women who start estrogen replacement therapy, about one-half discontinue it within six months.

3. Forty-three percent of patients do not take long-term medications as prescribed.

4. Thirty-eight percent of patients fail to follow short-term treatment plans (such as taking antibiotics).

5. Up to 21 percent of prescriptions given to patients are never filled.

6. Seventy-five percent of patients do not follow lifestyle recommendations (diet, exercise, etc.).

7. Fifty percent of patients in post-heart attack rehabilitation programs abandon them within a year.

8. Only 30 percent of patients follow dietary recommendations after one year.

9. Of patients taking digitalis for heart failure, only 10 percent have their prescriptions filled often enough to be receiving the proper dose.

10. About half of all patients leave the doctor's office not knowing what they have been advised to do.

11. One study found that patients with heart disease who took less than 80 percent of the prescribed medication (beta-blockers) had four times the number of cardiac events (heart attacks and strokes) as those who were fully adherent.

12. Up to 20 percent of patients do not present their prescriptions to a pharmacy within one month of issue.

Many of these above listed facts were noted in the September 1994 Johns Hopkins Medical Letter. They explain why many physicians feel frustrated with the practice of medicine.

Adult patients are not compliant for a variety of reasons, discontinuing medications on their own because of:

- Real or suspected side effects
- Drug costs
- Uncertainty of effectiveness
- Vacations
- Confusion about dose or time of dose
- Just plain forgetfulness

Doctors, at times, contribute to the problem by:

- Not giving patients clear directions
- Not warning patients about significant or bothersome side effects
- Making dose or time schedules too complicated
- Not recognizing medication cost factors
- Failing to instruct patients as to the purpose and importance of medications

Physicians may at times fail to recognize a drug's side effect that becomes manifest when added to other drugs on a patient's program. Patients, on the other hand, take supplements, non-prescription drugs, herbs, and various other pills with unknown components in varied forms and dosages without telling their physicians. Some of these drugs can be harmful in and of themselves, in combination with other medications patients take on their own (e.g., aspirin, sinus medications, etc.), or when used alongside prescribed medications.

Recommendations

1. Know the medications you take and why you are taking them.

2. Ask your doctor about side effects of prescribed medications you are given.

3. Have your doctor write down instructions.

4. Keep a list of your medications and instructions with you at all times.

5. Ask your doctor about less expensive alternatives for expensive medications.

6. Inform your doctor about suspected medication side effects.

7. Take a list of your current medications at least yearly to your doctor and do so more often if you take numerous medications.

8. Take a spouse, relative, or friend with you to your doctor when you discuss confusing or complex treatment programs.

9. If possible, choose a single pharmacy and personal pharmacist who is interested in providing information to you as well as in filling your prescriptions.

10. A pill container divided into daily compartments holding each day's medications is helpful for the elderly.

Further Reading

The Johns Hopkins Medical Letter, Health After 50. September, 1994.

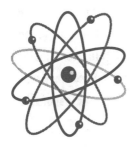

Where the Mind Leads the Body Will Follow

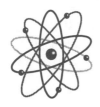

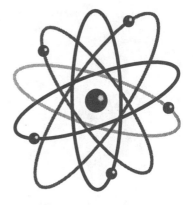

I could not at any age be content to take my place in a corner by the fireside and simply look on. Life was meant to be lived. Curiosity must be kept alive. The fatal thing is rejection. One must never, for whatever reason, turn his back on life.

-Eleanor Roosevelt

Current scientific data provide a great deal of information on extending length and quality of life. Better yet, the things we must do to achieve added years are not so difficult or unpleasant that we would need to wonder if they are worth the effort. In fact, many of the principles of life extension were taught to us by our mothers, who admonished:

- Don't smoke.
- Eat your fruits and vegetables.
- All that greasy food isn't good for you.
- Don't sit around. Go out and play!
- Let's do some work around here.
- You're getting fat. Don't eat so much junk.
- Why do you have to drink (alcohol)?
- Drink your milk.
- Don't ever let me hear that you are using drugs.
- Get your sleep. Don't stay up all night.
- What did the doctor tell you to do?
- Why don't you find yourself some nice friends?
- Buckle-up.

In this era of great medical advancements, physicians feel compelled to modify somewhat the wonderful words of wisdom passed on to us by our mothers. They might rephrase the messages to say:

- Don't smoke.
- Eat at least five servings of fruits and vegetables each day.
- Eat a diet low in fat, especially saturated fat and cholesterol.
- Know your blood pressure and be sure that it is normal.
- Exercise. Walk (or do some other aerobic activity) at least one-half hour each day.
- Keep your weight as close as possible to ideal for your height and build.

○ Work closely with your physician on cancer screening, blood pressure control, immunizations, and vitamin, mineral, and estrogen supplements.

○ Avoid more than one or two alcoholic drinks daily.

○ Stay away from all illicit drugs.

○ Maintain a supportive social network.

If you follow this advice, either your mother's or your physician's, and you don't lengthen your life, notify the authors of this book and they will cheerfully refund your money.

Further Reading/References

Several outstanding sources of information on topics related to life extension are available for those interested in reading further on the subject.

BOOKS

Guide to Clinical Preventive Services, Report of the U.S. Preventive Services Task Force, 2nd ed. Williams & Wilkins 1996.

Healthy People 2000, Midcourse Review and 1995 Revisions. U.S. Department of Health and Human Services, Public Health Service.

Living Well, Staying Well: Big Health Rewards from Small Lifestyle Changes. American Heart Association and American Cancer Society, Times Books 1996.

Barrett S, Herbert V: *The Vitamin Pushers.* Prometheus Books, Amherst, N.Y. 1994.

Dietary Guidelines for Americans, 4th ed. U.S. Department of Agriculture and the U.S. Department of Health and Human Services 1994.

OTHER

Authoritative, ongoing information on subjects related to life extension can be found in the following sources:

Harvard Health Letter, 164 Longwood Ave., Boston, MA 02115.

Harvard Heart Letter, 164 Longwood Ave., Boston, MA 02115.

The Johns Hopkins Medical Letter: Health after 50, 550 North Broadway, Suite 1100, Johns Hopkins, Baltimore, MD 21205-2011.

Mayo Clinic Health Letter, 200 First Street SW, Rochester, MN 55905.

Nutrition and the M.D.: PM, Inc., 7100 Hayvenhurst #107, Van Nuys, CA 91406.